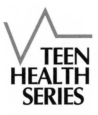

**TEEN
HEALTH
SERIES**

First Edition

Abuse and Violence Information for Teens

Health Tips about the Causes and Consequences of Abusive and Violent Behavior

*Including Facts about the Types of Abuse
and Violence, the Warning Signs of Abusive
and Violent Behavior, Health Concerns of Victims,
and Getting Help and Staying Safe*

◆

Edited by Sandra Augustyn Lawton

Omnigraphics

P.O. Box 31-1640, Detroit, MI 48231

Bibliographic Note

Because this page cannot legibly accommodate all the copyright notices, the Bibliographic Note portion of the Preface constitutes an extension of the copyright notice.

Edited by Sandra Augustyn Lawton

Teen Health Series

Karen Bellenir, *Managing Editor*
David A. Cooke, M.D., *Medical Consultant*
Elizabeth Collins, *Research and Permissions Coordinator*
Cherry Stockdale, *Permissions Assistant*
EdIndex, Services for Publishers, *Indexers*

* * *

Omnigraphics, Inc.

Matthew P. Barbour, *Senior Vice President*
Kay Gill, *Vice President—Directories*
Kevin M. Hayes, *Operations Manager*

* * *_

Peter E. Ruffner, *Publisher*

Copyright © 2008 Omnigraphics, Inc.

ISBN 978-0-7808-1008-2

Library of Congress Cataloging-in-Publication Data

Abuse and violence information for teens : health tips about the causes and consequences of abusive and violent behavior, including facts about the types of abuse and violence, the warning signs of abusive and violent behavior, health concerns of victims, and getting help and staying safe / edited by Sandra Augustyn Lawton.
    p. cm. -- (Teen health series)
    Summary: "Provides basic consumer health information for teens about risk factors, consequences, and prevention of various types of abuse and violence. Includes index, resource information and recommendations for further reading"--Provided by publisher.
    Includes bibliographical references and index.
    ISBN 978-0-7808-1008-2 (hardcover : alk. paper) 1. Youth and violence--United States. 2. Youth and violence--United States--Prevention. I. Lawton, Sandra Augustyn.
    HQ799.2.V56A28 2007
    362.76--dc22
                                                                    2007033611

Table of Contents

Part Two: Violence And The Teen Experience

Part Three: Recognizing And Treating The Consequences Of Abuse And Violence

Part Four: Prevention, Staying Safe, And Your Legal Rights As A Victim

Part Five: If You Need More Information

Preface

About This Book

Teens experience violence in many forms, including bullying, fighting, hazing, dating violence, sexual abuse, domestic violence, and even homicide. In 2003, more than 5,500 young people between the ages of 10 and 24 were murdered, 82 percent with a firearm. Although media coverage often focuses on shootings, other types of violence impact greater numbers of teens. In fact, according to statistics for 2004, more than 750,000 young people were treated in emergency rooms for a variety of injuries sustained as a result of violence, and the numbers of teens who suffer without receiving urgent medical care remain uncounted. The physical and emotional scars resulting from these experiences can endure for a lifetime.

Abuse and Violence Information for Teens discusses contributing factors and warning signs for the most commonly experienced types of abuse and violence. Facts about seeking medical care and mental health services for the physical and emotional consequences are also included. A section on prevention and safety suggests ways teens can help prevent violence and offers guidelines for staying out of harm's way. In addition, information about victims' rights is provided, and the book concludes with a resource section featuring statistical data, directories of organizations and agencies able to offer assistance, and suggestions for additional reading.

How To Use This Book

This book is divided into parts and chapters. Parts focus on broad areas of interest; chapters are devoted to single topics within a part.

Part One: Types Of Abuse provides information on domestic violence, child abuse, sibling abuse, sexual abuse, incest, stalking, and sexual harassment. It also discusses the role new technologies play in child pornography and sexual exploitation.

Part Two: Violence And The Teen Experience begins with a discussion regarding possible risk factors and warning signs for youth violence, including conduct disorders, media and video game violence, animal abuse, and substance abuse. It continues with facts about forms of violence teens often encounter. These include dating violence, bullying, hazing, and gang-related activity. The part concludes with facts about self-injury and suicide.

Part Three: Recognizing And Treating The Consequences Of Abuse And Violence explains the aftermath and repercussions of traumatic experiences. It explains what to do after a sexual assault and discusses the potential long-term effects of child abuse and neglect. It also provides facts about depression, posttraumatic stress disorder, and other mental health issues related to the experience of abuse and violence.

Part Four: Prevention, Staying Safe, And Your Legal Rights As A Victim discusses what can be done to prevent abuse and violence and gives helpful information about how to stay safe in an abusive or violent situation. It concludes with facts about a victim's legal rights.

Part Five: If You Need More Information includes a statistical summary of abuse and violence, resource directories, and suggestions for further reading.

Bibliographic Note

This volume contains documents and excerpts from publications issued by the following government agencies: Centers for Disease Control and Prevention (CDC); Child Welfare Information Gateway; Department of Justice (DOJ); Federal Emergency Management Agency (FEMA); National Center for Post-Traumatic Stress Disorder; National Criminal Justice Reference Service; National Institute of Mental Health (NIMH); National Youth Violence Prevention Resource Center; National Women's Health Information Center (NWHIC); Office of the Surgeon General (U.S.), Substance Abuse and Mental

Health Services Administration (SAMHSA); and the U.S. Department of Agriculture (USDA).

In addition, this volume contains copyrighted documents and articles produced by the following organizations and individuals: About, Inc.; Advocates for Youth; American Geriatrics Society Foundation for Health in Aging; American Psychological Association; Childhelp; James Chandler, M.D.; Domestic Violence and Incest Resource Centre; Family Violence Prevention Fund; Helpguide.org; Humane Society of the United States; National Association for Children of Alcoholics; National Center for Victims of Crime; Nemours Foundation; Rape, Abuse and Incest National Network; *Science News for Kids*; Sidran Institute; StopHazing.org; UNICEF; University of Colorado; University of Michigan Health System; and the WebMD Corporation.

Full citation information is provided on the first page of each chapter. Every effort has been made to secure all necessary rights to reprint the copyrighted material. If any omissions have been made, please contact Omnigraphics to make corrections for future editions.

The photograph on the front cover is from Design Pics/Photosearch.com.

Acknowledgements

In addition to the organizations listed above, special thanks are due to the *Teen Health Series* research and permissions coordinator, Elizabeth Collins, and to its managing editor, Karen Bellenir.

About the *Teen Health Series*

At the request of librarians serving today's young adults, the *Teen Health Series* was developed as a specially focused set of volumes within Omnigraphics' *Health Reference Series*. Each volume deals comprehensively with a topic selected according to the needs and interests of people in middle school and high school.

Teens seeking preventive guidance, information about disease warning signs, medical statistics, and risk factors for health problems will find answers to their questions in the *Teen Health Series*. The *Series*, however, is not intended to serve as a tool for diagnosing illness, in prescribing treatments, or as a substitute for the physician/patient relationship. All people concerned about medical symptoms or the possibility of disease are encouraged to seek professional care from an appropriate health care provider.

If there is a topic you would like to see addressed in a future volume of the *Teen Health Series*, please write to:

Editor
Teen Health Series
Omnigraphics, Inc.
P.O. Box 31-1640
Detroit, MI 48231

A Note about Spelling and Style

Teen Health Series editors use *Stedman's Medical Dictionary* as an authority for questions related to the spelling of medical terms and the *Chicago Manual of Style* for questions related to grammatical structures, punctuation, and other editorial concerns. Consistent adherence is not always possible, however, because the individual volumes within the *Series* include many documents from a wide variety of different producers and copyright holders, and the editor's primary goal is to present material from each source as accurately as is possible following the terms specified by each document's producer. This sometimes means that information in different chapters or sections may follow other guidelines and alternate spelling authorities. For example, occasionally a copyright holder may require that eponymous terms be shown in possessive forms (Crohn's disease *vs.* Crohn disease) or that British spelling norms be retained (leukaemia *vs.* leukemia).

Locating Information within the *Teen Health Series*

The *Teen Health Series* contains a wealth of information about a wide variety of medical topics. As the *Series* continues to grow in size and scope, locating the precise information needed by a specific student may become more challenging. To address this concern, information about books within the *Teen Health Series* is included in *A Contents Guide to the Health Reference Series*. The *Contents Guide* presents an extensive list of more than 13,000 diseases, treatments, and other topics of general interest compiled from the Tables of Contents and major index headings from the books of the *Teen Health Series* and *Health Reference Series*. To access *A Contents Guide to the Health Reference Series*, visit www.healthreferenceseries.com.

Our Advisory Board

We would like to thank the following advisory board members for providing guidance to the development of this *Series*:

Dr. Lynda Baker, Associate Professor of Library and Information Science, Wayne State University, Detroit, MI

Nancy Bulgarelli, William Beaumont Hospital Library, Royal Oak, MI

Karen Imarisio, Bloomfield Township Public Library, Bloomfield Township, MI

Karen Morgan, Mardigian Library, University of Michigan-Dearborn, Dearborn, MI

Rosemary Orlando, St. Clair Shores Public Library, St. Clair Shores, MI

Medical Consultant

Medical consultation services are provided to the *Teen Health Series* editors by David A. Cooke, M.D. Dr. Cooke is a graduate of Brandeis University, and he received his M.D. degree from the University of Michigan. He completed residency training at the University of Wisconsin Hospital and Clinics. He is board-certified in internal medicine. Dr. Cooke currently works as part of the University of Michigan Health System and practices in Ann Arbor, MI. In his free time, he enjoys writing, science fiction, and spending time with his family.

Part One

Types Of Abuse

Chapter 1

Abuse In Families: An Overview

Amy's finger was so swollen that she couldn't get her ring off. She didn't think her finger was broken because she could still bend it. It had been a week since her dad had grabbed her hand and then shoved her into the wall, but her finger still hurt a lot. She was so embarrassed that she didn't tell anyone. Amy hated the way her dad called her lots of names—and accused her of all sorts of things she didn't do—especially after he had been drinking. It made her feel awful. She wished he would stop, but didn't feel very hopeful that anything would change.

What Is Abuse?

Abuse in families can take many forms. It may be physical, sexual, emotional, verbal, or a combination of any or all of those. Neglect—when parents don't take care of the basic needs of the children who depend on them—can be a form of abuse.

Family violence can affect anyone, regardless of religion, color, or social standing. It happens in both wealthy and poor families and in single-parent or two-parent households. Sometimes parents abuse each other, which can be hard for a child to witness. Some parents abuse their children by using

About This Chapter: Information in this chapter is from "Abuse." This information was provided by TeensHealth, one of the largest resources online for medically reviewed health information written for teens, kids, and parents. For more articles like this one, visit www.TeensHealth.org, or www.KidsHealth.org. © 2004 The Nemours Foundation.

People who are experiencing abuse often feel weird or alone. But they're not. No one deserves to be abused. Getting help and support is an important first step to change the situation. Many teens who have experienced abuse find that painful emotions may linger even after the abuse stops. Working with a therapist is one way for a person to sort through the complicated feelings and reactions that being abused creates, and the process can help to rebuild feelings of safety, confidence, and self-esteem.

Chapter 2

What Is Domestic Violence?

What is domestic violence?

Domestic violence is defined as the use or threat of use of physical, emotional, verbal, or sexual abuse with the intent of instilling fear, intimidating, and controlling behavior. Domestic violence occurs within the context of an intimate relationship and may continue after the relationship has ended. The types of domestic violence are as follows:

- **Physical Abuse:** Verbal threats of violence, pushing, shoving, hitting, slapping, punching, biting, kicking, holding down, pinning against the wall, choking, throwing objects, breaking objects, punching walls, driving recklessly to scare, blocking exits, using weapons

- **Emotional/Verbal Abuse:** Name calling, coercion and threats, criticizing, yelling, humiliating, isolating, economic abuse (controlling finances, preventing victim from working), threatening to hurt children or pets, stalking

- **Sexual Abuse:** Unwanted touching, sexual name calling, false accusations of sexual infidelity, forced sex, unwanted pregnancy, sexually transmitted diseases, HIV transmission

About This Chapter: Information in this chapter is excerpted from "Domestic Violence," by Michelle Rice, Ph.D., National Center for Posttraumatic Stress Disorder, United States Department of Veterans Affairs, February 2007.

Researchers in the field of domestic violence have compiled characteristics of batterers, which can be utilized to predict the likelihood of battering. The more characteristics present in a person, the greater the likelihood of battering. The most predictive indicators are as follows:

- history of past battering

- threats of violence

- breaking objects

- use of force during arguments

The following are also warning signs:

- unreasonable jealousy

- controlling behavior

- quick involvement in the relationship

- verbal abuse, blaming others for problems

- cruelty to children and animals

- abrupt mood changes

> **♣ It's A Fact!!**
> Domestic violence is the most frequent cause of serious injury to women, more than car accidents, muggings, and stranger rapes combined.

What is the prevalence of domestic violence?

It is very difficult to estimate the rate of domestic violence because the majority of victims never disclose that they are involved in partner violence. It is estimated that, regarding violent behavior toward females within the context of an intimate relationship, only 20% of all rapes, 25% of all physical assaults, and 50% of all stalking are ever reported to the police. Victims may be reluctant to come forward for a variety of reasons. First, they may fear retaliation from their partner. They may have been directly threatened that if they tell anyone, they will be killed, or they may just fear the worst. Second, there is shame associated with choosing a partner who could be violent, and there is shame associated with staying with a violent partner. Finally, some victims may have tried to seek help from the police, the courts, or others and been dissatisfied with the help they received. The following statistics shed light on the prevalence of domestic violence in the United States:

- 20–30% of American women will be physically abused by a partner at least once in their lifetimes

- 1.3 million women and 834,732 men are physically assaulted by an intimate partner annually

- 201,394 women are forcibly raped by an intimate partner annually

- 11% of women in homosexual relationships and 23% of men in homosexual relationships report being raped, physically assaulted, and/or stalked by an intimate partner

- 503,485 women and 185,496 men are stalked by an intimate partner annually

- 1–25% of all pregnant women are battered during pregnancy

- 30–40% of women's emergency room visits are for injuries due to domestic violence

- 30% of women killed in the U.S. are killed by their husbands or boyfriends

- 50% of men who assaulted their female partners also assaulted their children

- 3.3 million children witness domestic violence each year

What are the dynamics of an abusive relationship?

Research focusing on the dynamics of abusive relationships has resulted in several ways of understanding the interactions between the batterer and the victim. The first conceptualization is that of the "cycle of violence" consisting of three stages: the tension building stage (tension in the relationship gradually increases over time); the acute battering stage (tension erupts, resulting in threats or use of violence and abuse); and the honeymoon stage (the batterer may be apologetic and remorseful and promise not to be abusive again). The cycle continues throughout the relationship with the honeymoon stage becoming shorter and the episodes of battering becoming more frequent or more severe. The honeymoon stage reinforces the victim's hope that the batterer will change and contributes to the victim staying in the relationship.

The concept of "traumatic bonding" has also been developed to explain the dynamics of domestic violence relationships. Essentially, strong emotional connections develop between the victim and the perpetrator during the abusive relationship. These emotional ties develop due to the imbalance of power between the batterer and the victim and because the treatment is intermittently good and bad. In terms of the power imbalance, as the abuser gains more power, the abused individual feels worse about him- or herself, is less able to protect him- or herself, and is less competent. The abused person therefore becomes increasingly dependent on the abuser. The second key factor in traumatic bonding is the intermittent and unpredictable abuse. While this may sound counterintuitive, the abuse is offset by an increase in positive behaviors such as attention, gifts, and promises. The abused individual also feels relief that the abuse has ended. Thus, there is intermittent reinforcement for the behavior, which is difficult to extinguish and serves instead to strengthen the bond between the abuser and the individual being abused.

Finally, abusive relationship dynamics can also be understood through the concepts of "approach and avoidance." The mix of pros (love and economic support) and cons (fear and humiliation) present in the battering relationship leads to ambivalence on the part of the victim. The victim is likely to want to approach the positives in the relationship but avoid the abuse. This struggle between wanting to keep the relationship and wanting to remain safe makes it difficult to decide whether to leave or stay in the relationship.

> ♣ **It's A Fact!!**
> On average, women leave and return to an abusive relationship five times before permanently leaving the relationship.

What are the effects of domestic violence?

Domestic violence has wide ranging and sometimes long-term effects on victims. The effects can be both physical and psychological and can impact the direct victim as well as any children who witness parental violence.

The physical health effects of domestic violence are varied. Victims may experience physical injury (lacerations, bruises, broken bones, head injuries, internal bleeding), chronic pelvic pain, abdominal and gastrointestinal complaints, frequent vaginal and urinary tract infections, sexually transmitted diseases, and HIV. Victims may also experience pregnancy-related problems. Women who are battered during pregnancy are at higher risk for poor weight gain, pre-term labor, miscarriage, low infant birth weight, and injury to, or death of, the fetus.

There are also many psychological effects of domestic violence. Depression remains the foremost response with 60% of battered women reporting depression. In addition, battered women are at greater risk for suicide attempts with 25% of suicide attempts by Caucasian women and 50% of suicide attempts by African American women preceded by abuse.

Along with depression, domestic violence victims may also experience posttraumatic stress disorder (PTSD), which is characterized by symptoms such as flashbacks, intrusive imagery, nightmares, anxiety, emotional numbing, insomnia, hyper-vigilance, and avoidance of traumatic triggers.

Children may develop behavioral or emotional difficulties after experiencing physical abuse in the context of domestic violence or after witnessing parental abuse. Children's responses to the violence may vary from aggression to withdrawal to physical complaints. In addition, children may develop symptoms of depression, anxiety, or PTSD.

How are the effects of domestic violence treated?

Psychological treatment for victims and perpetrators can be helpful in the aftermath of domestic violence. For battered women, a feminist therapy approach is recommended in which traditional gender roles are challenged and empowerment of the victim is a primary focus. Individual therapy for victims of domestic violence should begin with a primary focus on safety, particularly if the woman is currently in an abusive relationship. The therapist should assess the current level of dangerousness and lethality in the relationship based on the following factors concerning the batterer: threats of homicide or suicide, possession of weapons, acute depression, alcohol/drug use, history of pet abuse, and level of rage. The presence of these factors increases the level of potential lethality in the batterer.

In addition to assessing lethality, the individual therapist should develop a safety plan with the victim. A safety plan may contain a strategy for how to leave a dangerous situation; the preparation of a safety kit (clothing, medications, keys, money, copies of important documents) to be kept either near an exit route or at a trusted friend's house; and arrangements for shelter (made without the batterer's knowledge of the location).

Once lethality and safety have been addressed, the longer-term goals of treatment for the battered woman can be addressed. These goals include helping the woman identify the impact of abuse on her life and helping her work toward empowerment. Victims can be empowered by regaining their independence and reconnecting with supports and resources that may have been cut off due to the isolation of domestic violence. In addition, the victim's children may need their own treatment to address their responses to witnessing or experiencing abuse.

For some victims, additional treatment may be needed to target symptoms of depression, PTSD, substance abuse, or other disorders found to occur in the presence of domestic violence.

Batterers can also benefit from treatment, although it remains unclear exactly how effective treatment is in breaking the cycle of batterers' violence. Batterers benefit most from batterer treatment programs, which in part focus on identifying what domestic violence is. These programs also focus on helping batterers develop a sense of personal responsibility for one's actions and for stopping the violence. Batterers can also be treated in individual therapy, but the focus of treatment must be on the violence. While some batterers and victims may seek to engage in couple's therapy to address the abuse in their relationship, couple's therapy is not recommended while violence is occurring in the relationship. In addition, it is recommended that each member of the couple complete their individual treatment first, before beginning any couple's therapy.

Chapter 3

Child Abuse

Physical Abuse

Generally, physical abuse is characterized by physical injury such as bruises and fractures that result from punching, beating, kicking, biting, shaking, throwing, stabbing, choking, burning, or hitting with a hand, stick, strap, or other object.

Although an injury resulting from physical abuse is not accidental, the parent or caregiver may not have intended to hurt the child. The injury may have resulted from severe discipline, including injurious spanking, or physical punishment that is inappropriate to the child's age or condition. The injury may be the result of a single episode or repeated episodes and can range in severity from minor marks and bruising to death.

As Howard Dubowitz, a leading researcher in the field explains: "While cultural practices are generally respected, if the injury or harm is significant,

About This Chapter: Information in this chapter is from "Physical Abuse," July 2006, "Signs of Physical Abuse*," August 2006, "Emotional Abuse," July 2006, "Signs of Emotional Abuse*," August 2006, "Sexual Abuse," July 2006, "Signs of Sexual Abuse*," August 2006, "Physical Neglect," July 2006, "Emotional Neglect," July 2006, "Educational Neglect," July 2006, and "Signs of Neglect*," August 2006; Child Welfare Information Gateway (www.childwelfare.gov), Children's Bureau, Administration for Children, Youth and Families, U.S. Department of Health and Human Services. *This information was adapted, with permission, from "Recognizing Child Abuse: What Parents Should Know." Prevent Child Abuse America. © 2003.

professionals typically work with parents to discourage harmful behavior and suggest preferable alternatives."

Signs Of Physical Abuse

The presence of a single sign does not prove child abuse is occurring in a family; however, when these signs appear repeatedly or in combination, you should take a closer look at the situation and consider the possibility of child abuse.

Consider the possibility of physical abuse in the following situations:

- The child has unexplained burns, bites, bruises, broken bones, or black eyes.

- The child has fading bruises or other marks noticeable after an absence from school.

- The child seems frightened of the parents and protests or cries when it is time to go home.

- The child shrinks at the approach of adults.

- The child reports injury by a parent or another adult caregiver.

♣ **It's A Fact!!**
Of the estimated 872,000 children who were found to be victims of maltreatment in 2004, 17.5 percent were physically abused.

Source: Excerpted from "Physical Abuse," July 2006, Child Welfare Information Gateway.

Consider the possibility of physical abuse when the following is true of a parent or other adult caregiver:

- offers conflicting, unconvincing, or no explanation for the child's injury

- describes the child as "evil" or in some other very negative way

- uses harsh physical discipline with the child

- has a history of abuse as a child

Note: This information was adapted, with permission, from *Recognizing Child Abuse: What Parents Should Know*. Prevent Child Abuse America. © 2003.

Emotional Abuse

Psychological maltreatment, also known as emotional abuse, refers to "a repeated pattern of caregiver behavior or extreme incident(s) that convey to children that they are worthless, flawed, unloved, unwanted, endangered, or only of value in meeting another's needs."

Summarizing research and expert opinion, Stuart N. Hart, Ph.D. and Marla R. Brassard, PhD., present six categories of psychological maltreatment. They are as follows:

- spurning (e.g., belittling, hostile rejecting, ridiculing)

- terrorizing (e.g., threatening violence against a child, placing a child in a recognizably dangerous situation)

- isolating (e.g., confining the child, placing unreasonable limitations on the child's freedom of movement, restricting the child from social interactions)

- exploiting or corrupting (e.g., modeling antisocial behavior such as criminal activities, encouraging prostitution, permitting substance abuse)

- denying emotional responsiveness (e.g., ignoring the child's attempts to interact, failing to express affection)

- mental health, medical, and educational neglect (e.g., refusing to allow, or failing to provide treatment, for serious mental health or medical problems, ignoring the need for services for serious educational needs)

♣ It's A Fact!!
Of the estimated 872,000 children who were found to be victims of maltreatment in 2004, 7.0 percent were emotionally or psychologically maltreated.

Source: Excerpted from " Emotional Abuse," July 2006, Child Welfare Information Gateway.

Signs Of Emotional Abuse

Consider the possibility of emotional maltreatment in the following situations:

- The child shows extremes in behavior such as overly compliant or demanding behavior, extreme passivity, or aggression.

- The child is either inappropriately adult (parenting other children, for example) or inappropriately infantile (frequently rocking or head-banging, for example)

- The child is delayed in physical or emotional development.

- The child has attempted suicide.

- The child reports a lack of attachment to the parent.

Consider the possibility of emotional maltreatment when the parent or other adult caregiver does the following:

- constantly blames, belittles, or berates the child

- is unconcerned about the child and refuses to consider offers of help for the child's problems

- overtly rejects the child

Note: This information was adapted, with permission, from *Recognizing Child Abuse: What Parents Should Know*. Prevent Child Abuse America. © 2003.

Sexual Abuse

Child sexual abuse generally refers to sexual acts, sexually motivated behaviors, or sexual exploitation involving children. Child sexual abuse includes a wide range of behaviors such as the following:

- oral, anal, or genital penile penetration

- anal or genital digital or other penetration

- genital contact with no intrusion

- fondling of a child's breasts or buttocks

- indecent exposure

- inadequate or inappropriate supervision of a child's voluntary sexual activities

- use of a child in prostitution, pornography, internet crimes, or other sexually exploitative activities

Sexual abuse includes both touching offenses (fondling or sexual intercourse) and non-touching offenses (exposing a child to pornographic materials) and can involve varying degrees of violence and emotional trauma. The most commonly reported cases involve incest, or sexual abuse occurring among family members, including those in biological families, adoptive families, and stepfamilies. Incest most often occurs within a father-daughter relationship; however, mother-son, father-son, and sibling-sibling incest also occurs. Sexual abuse is also sometimes committed by other relatives or caretakers.

♣ It's A Fact!!

Of the estimated 872,000 children who were found to be victims of maltreatment in 2004, 9.7 percent were sexually abused.

Source: Excerpted from "Sexual Abuse," July 2006, Child Welfare Information Gateway.

Signs Of Sexual Abuse

Consider the possibility of sexual abuse in the following situations:

- The child has difficulty walking or sitting.

- The child suddenly refuses to change for gym or to participate in physical activities.

- The child reports nightmares or bedwetting.

- The child experiences a sudden change in appetite.

- The child demonstrates bizarre, sophisticated, or unusual sexual knowledge or behavior.

- The child becomes pregnant or contracts a venereal disease, particularly if under age 14.

- The child runs away.

- The child reports sexual abuse by a parent or another adult caregiver.

Consider the possibility of sexual abuse when the following is true of a parent or other adult caregiver:

- He or she is unduly protective of the child or severely limits the child's contact with other children, especially of the opposite sex.

- He or she is secretive and isolated.

- He or she is jealous or controlling with family members.

Note: This information was adapted, with permission, from *Recognizing Child Abuse: What Parents Should Know*. Prevent Child Abuse America. © 2003.

Physical Neglect

The Department of Health and Human Services' Third National Incidence Study of Child Abuse and Neglect (NIS-3) defines physical neglect as any of the following:

- **Refusal of Health Care:** Failure to provide or allow needed care in accordance with recommendations of a competent health care professional for a physical injury, illness, medical condition, or impairment.

- **Delay In Health Care:** Failure to seek timely and appropriate medical care for a serious health problem that any reasonable layperson would have recognized as needing professional medical attention.

- **Abandonment:** Desertion of a child without arranging for reasonable care and supervision.

- **Expulsion:** Other blatant refusals of custody such as permanent or indefinite expulsion of a child from the home without adequate arrangement for care by others or refusal to accept custody of a returned runaway.

- **Inadequate Supervision:** Leaving a child unsupervised or inadequately supervised for extended periods of time or allowing the child to remain away from home overnight without knowing or attempting to determine the child's whereabouts.

- **Other Physical Neglect:** May include inadequate nutrition, clothing, or hygiene; conspicuous inattention to avoidable hazards in the home; and other forms of reckless disregard for the child's safety and welfare (e.g., driving with the child while intoxicated, leaving a young child unattended in a car).

Munchausen Syndrome By Proxy

Munchausen syndrome is a psychological disorder in which the patient fabricates the symptoms of disease or injury in order to undergo medical tests, hospitalization, or even medical or surgical treatment. To command medical attention, patients with Munchausen syndrome may intentionally injure themselves or induce illness in themselves. In cases of Munchausen syndrome by proxy, a parent or caretaker suffering from Munchausen syndrome attempts to bring medical attention to themselves by injuring or inducing illness in their children. The parent then may try to resuscitate the child or to have paramedics or hospital personnel save the child. The following scenarios are common occurrences in these cases:

- The child's caretaker repeatedly brings the child for medical care or calls paramedics for alleged problems that cannot be medically documented.

- The child only experiences "seizures" or "respiratory arrest" when the caretaker is there—never in the presence of neutral third parties or in the hospital.

- When the child is hospitalized, the caretaker turns off the life support equipment, causing the child to stop breathing, and then turns everything back on and summons help.

- The caretaker induces illness by introducing a mild irritant or poison into the child's body.

Source: Excerpted from "Battered Child Syndrome: Investigating Physical Abuse and Homicide," Office of Juvenile Justice and Delinquency Prevention, a component of the Office of Justice Programs, U.S. Department of Justice, December 2002.

Emotional Neglect

The Department of Health and Human Services' Third National Incidence Study of Child Abuse and Neglect (NIS-3) defines emotional neglect as any of the following:

- **Inadequate Nurturing Or Affection:** Marked inattention to the child's needs for affection, emotional support, or attention.

- **Chronic Or Extreme Spouse Abuse:** Exposure of the child to chronic or extreme spouse abuse or other domestic violence.

- **Permitted Drug Or Alcohol Abuse:** Encouragement or permission of drug or alcohol use by the child.

- **Permitted Other Maladaptive Behavior:** Encouragement or permission of other maladaptive behavior (e.g., chronic delinquency, severe assault) under circumstances where the parent or caregiver has reason to be aware of the existence and seriousness of the problem but does not intervene.

- **Refusal Of Psychological Care:** Refusal to allow needed and available treatment for a child's emotional or behavioral impairment or problem in accordance with a competent professional recommendation.

- **Delay In Psychological Care:** Failure to seek or provide needed treatment for a child's emotional or behavioral impairment or problem that any reasonable layperson would have recognized as needing professional psychological attention (e.g., suicide attempt).

Educational Neglect

The Department of Health and Human Services' Third National Incidence Study of Child Abuse and Neglect (NIS-3) defines educational neglect as any of the following:

- **Permitted Chronic Truancy:** Habitual absenteeism from school averaging at least five days a month if the parent or guardian is informed of the problem and does not attempt to intervene.

- **Failure To Enroll Or Other Truancy:** Failure to register or enroll a child of mandatory school age, causing the child to miss at least one month of school, or a pattern of keeping a school-aged child home without valid reasons.

- **Inattention To Special Education Need:** Refusal to allow, or failure to obtain, recommended remedial education services or neglect in obtaining, or following through with treatment, for a child's diagnosed learning disorder or other special education need without reasonable cause.

Signs Of Neglect

The presence of a single sign does not prove child neglect is occurring in a family; however, when these signs appear repeatedly or in combination, you should take a closer look at the situation and consider the possibility of child neglect.

Consider the possibility of neglect in the following situations:

- The child is frequently absent from school.
- The child begs or steals food or money.
- The child lacks needed medical or dental care, immunizations, or glasses.
- The child is consistently dirty and has severe body odor.
- The child lacks sufficient clothing for the weather.
- The child abuses alcohol or other drugs.
- The child states that there is no one at home to provide care.

Consider the possibility of neglect when the following is true of the parent or other adult caregiver:

- He or she appears to be indifferent to the child.
- He or she seems apathetic or depressed.
- He or she behaves irrationally or in a bizarre manner.
- He or she is abusing alcohol or other drugs.

Note: This information was adapted, with permission, from *Recognizing Child Abuse: What Parents Should Know.* Prevent Child Abuse America. © 2003.

Chapter 4

Children Of Addicted Parents: Increased Risks

Alcoholism and other drug addictions have genetic and environmental causes. Both have serious consequences for children who live in homes where parents are involved. More than 28 million Americans are children of alcoholics; nearly 11 million are under the age of 18. This figure is magnified by the countless number of others who are affected by parents who are impaired by other psychoactive drugs.

Alcoholism and other drug addictions tend to run in families. Children of addicted parents are more at risk for alcoholism and other drug abuse than are other children.

- Children of addicted parents are the highest risk group of children to become alcohol and drug abusers due to both genetic and family environment factors.

- Biological children of alcohol dependent parents who have been adopted continue to have an increased risk (2–9 fold) of developing alcoholism.

About This Chapter: Information in this chapter is from "Children of Addicted Parents: Important Facts." Reprinted with permission by the National Association for Children of Alcoholics, © 2003.

- Recent studies suggest a strong genetic component, particularly for early onset, of alcoholism in males. Sons of alcoholic fathers are at fourfold risk compared with the male offspring of non-alcoholic fathers.

- Use of substances by parents and their adolescent children is strongly correlated; generally, if parents take drugs, sooner or later their children will also.

> ♣ **It's A Fact!!**
> Adolescents who use drugs are more likely to have one or more parents who also use drugs.

- The influence of parental attitudes on a child's drug-taking behaviors may be as important as actual drug abuse by the parents. An adolescent who perceives that a parent is permissive about the use of drugs is more likely to use drugs.

Family interaction is defined by substance abuse or addiction in a family.

- Families affected by alcoholism report higher levels of conflict than do families with no alcoholism. Drinking is the primary factor in family disruption. The environment of children of alcoholics has been characterized by lack of parenting, poor home management, and lack of family communication skills, thereby effectively robbing children of alcoholic parents of modeling or training on parenting skills or family effectiveness.

- The following family problems have been frequently associated with families affected by alcoholism: increased family conflict; emotional or physical violence; decreased family cohesion; decreased family organization; increased family isolation; increased family stress including work problems, illness, marital strain, and financial problems; and frequent family moves.

- Addicted parents often lack the ability to provide structure or discipline in family life but simultaneously expect their children to be competent at a wide variety of tasks earlier than do non-substance-abusing parents.

- Sons of addicted fathers are the recipients of more detrimental discipline practices from their parents.

A relationship between parental addiction and child abuse has been documented in a large proportion of child abuse and neglect cases.

- Three of four (71.6%) child welfare professionals cite substance abuse as the top cause for the dramatic rise in child maltreatment since 1986.

- Most welfare professionals (79.6%) report that substance abuse causes, or contributes, to at least half of all cases of child maltreatment; 39.7% say it is a factor in over 75% of the cases.

- Children exposed prenatally to illicit drugs are 2 to 3 times more likely to be abused or neglected.

Children of drug-addicted parents are at higher risk for placement outside the home.

- Three of four child welfare professionals (75.7%) say that children of addicted parents are more likely to enter foster care, and 73% say that children of alcoholics stay longer in foster care than do other children.

- In one study, 79% of adolescent runaways and homeless youth reported alcohol use in the home, 53% reported problem drinking in the home, and 54% reported drug use in the home.

- Each year, approximately 11,900 infants are abandoned at birth or are kept at hospitals, 78% of whom are drug-exposed; the average daily cost for each of these babies is $460.

Children of addicted parents exhibit symptoms of depression and anxiety more than do children from non-addicted families.

- Children of addicted parents exhibit depression and depressive symptoms more frequently than do children from non-addicted families.

- Children of addicted parents are more likely to have anxiety disorders or to show anxiety symptoms.

> **♣ It's A Fact!!**
>
> In a sample of parents who significantly maltreat their children, alcohol abuse is specifically associated with physical maltreatment, while cocaine exhibits a specific relationship to sexual maltreatment.

- Children of addicted parents are at high risk for elevated rates of psychiatric and psychosocial dysfunction, as well as for alcoholism.

Children of addicted parents experience greater physical and mental health problems and higher health and welfare costs than do children from non-addicted families.

- Inpatient admission rates and average length of stay for children of alcoholics were 24% and 29% greater than for children of non-alcoholic parents. Substance abuse and other mental disorders were the most notable conditions among children of addicted parents.

- It is estimated that parental substance abuse and addiction are the chief cause in at least 70–90% of all child welfare spending. Using the more conservative 70% assessment, in 1998 substance abuse and addiction accounted for approximately $10 billion in federal, state, and local government spending simply to maintain child welfare systems.

- The economic costs associated with fetal alcohol syndrome were estimated at $1.9 billion for 1992.

- A sample of children hospitalized for psychiatric disorders demonstrated that more than 50% were children of addicted parents.

Children of addicted parents have a high rate of behavior problems.

- One study comparing children of alcoholics (aged 6–17 years) with children of psychiatrically healthy medical patients found that children of alcoholics had elevated rates of attention deficit hyperactivity disorder (ADHD) and oppositional defiant disorder (ODD) measured against the control group of children.

- Research on behavioral problems demonstrated by children of alcoholics has revealed some of the following traits: lack of empathy for other persons; decreased social adequacy and interpersonal adaptability; low self-esteem; and lack of control over the environment.

- Research has shown that children of addicted parents demonstrate behavioral characteristics and a temperament style that predispose them to future maladjustment.

Children of addicted parents score lower on tests measuring school achievement, and they exhibit other difficulties in school.

- Sons of addicted parents performed worse on all domains measuring school achievement using the Peabody Individual Achievement Test— Revised (PIAT-R) including general information, reading recognition, reading comprehension, total reading, mathematics, and spelling.

- In general, children of alcoholic parents do less well on academic measures. They also have higher rates of school absenteeism and are more likely to leave school, be retained, or be referred to the school psychologist than are children of nonalcoholic parents.

- In one study, 41% of addicted parents reported that at least one of their children repeated a grade in school, 19% were involved in truancy, and 30% had been suspended from school.

- Children of addicted parents, compared to children of non-addicted parents, were found at significant disadvantage on standard scores of arithmetic.

Maternal consumption of alcohol and other drugs during any time of pregnancy can cause birth defects or neurological deficits.

- Studies have shown that exposure to cocaine during fetal development may lead to subtle, but significant deficits later on, especially with behaviors that are crucial to success in the classroom such as blocking out distractions and concentrating for long periods.

- Cognitive performance is less affected by alcohol exposure in infants and children whose mothers stopped drinking in early pregnancy despite the mothers' resumption of alcohol use after giving birth.

♣ It's A Fact!!

Prenatal alcohol effects have been detected at moderate levels of alcohol consumption in nonalcoholic women. Even though a mother may not regularly abuse alcohol, her child may not be spared the effects of prenatal alcohol exposure.

Children of addicted parents may benefit from supportive adult efforts to help them.

- Children who coped effectively with the trauma of growing up in families affected by alcoholism often relied on the support of a non-alcoholic parent, stepparent, grandparent, teachers, and others.

- Children of addicted parents who rely on other supportive adults have increased autonomy and independence, stronger social skills, better ability to cope with difficult emotional experiences, and better day-to-day coping strategies.

- Group programs reduce feelings of isolation, shame, and guilt among children of alcoholics while capitalizing on the importance to adolescents of peer influence and mutual support.

- Competencies such as the ability to establish and maintain intimate relationships, express feelings, and solve problems can be improved by building the self-esteem and self-efficacy of children of alcoholics.

Chapter 5

Sibling Abuse

What is sibling abuse?

Sibling abuse is the physical, emotional, or sexual abuse of one sibling by another. The physical abuse can range from relatively mild forms of aggression occurring between siblings, such as pushing and shoving, to extremely violent behavior such as the use of weapons.

Often parents don't recognize the abuse for what it is. Typically, parents and society expect fights and other physical forms of aggression to occur among siblings. Because of this, sibling abuse often is not seen as a problem until serious injuries occur. Another factor is that in some cases, siblings may switch back and forth between the roles of abuser and victim.

Besides the immediate dangers of sibling abuse, the abuse can cause all kinds of problems on into adulthood. Being abused by a sibling can really mess up a person's life.

How common is sibling abuse?

Research shows that violence between siblings is quite common. In fact, it is probably even more common than child abuse (by parents) or spouse abuse. The most violent members of American families are the children.

Likewise, many researchers have estimated sibling incest to be much more common than parent-child incest. It seems that when abusive acts occur between siblings, they are often not perceived as abuse.

♣ **It's A Fact!!**
It has been estimated that three children in 100 are dangerously violent toward a brother or sister.

How do I identify abuse? What is the difference between sibling abuse and sibling rivalry?

At times, all siblings squabble and call each other mean names, and some young siblings will "play doctor". But here is the difference between typical sibling behavior and abuse: If one child is always the victim and the other child is always the aggressor, it is an abusive situation.

Some possible signs of sibling abuse are the following:

• One child always avoids their sibling.

• A child has changes in behavior, sleep patterns, eating habits, or has nightmares.

• A child acts out abuse in play.

• A child acts out sexually in inappropriate ways.

What are some of the risk factors for sibling abuse?

Much more research needs to be done to find out how and why sibling abuse happens. Some risk factors are as follows:

• Parents are not around much at home.

• Parents are not very involved in their children's lives or are emotionally unavailable to them.

• Parents accept sibling rivalry as part of family life rather than working to minimize it.

• Parents do not stop children when they are violent (they may assume it was accidental or part of a two-way fight).

- Parents increase competition among children by doing the following:

  - playing favorites

  - comparing children

  - labeling or typecasting children (even casting kids in positive roles is harmful)

- Parents have not taught children about sexuality and about personal safety.

- Parents and children are in denial that there is a problem.

- Children have inappropriate family roles; for example, they are burdened with too much care-taking responsibility for a younger sibling.

- Children are exposed to violence in the following ways:

  - in their family

  - in the media

  - among their peers

  - in their neighborhoods

- Children have been sexually abused or witnessed sexual abuse.

- Children have access to pornography.

♣ **It's A Fact!!**
Even less extreme sibling rivalry during childhood can create insecurity and poor self-image in adulthood. Sibling conflict does not have to be physically violent to take a long-lasting emotional toll. Emotional abuse, which includes teasing, name-calling, and isolation, can also do long-term damage.

Can sibling relationships have lasting effects into adulthood?

In the last few years, more research has been done on the lasting effects of early experiences with sisters and brothers. Siblings can have strong, sometimes long-lasting, effects on one another's emotional development as adults.

Research indicates that long-term effects of sibling abuse can include the following:

- depression, anxiety, and low self-esteem

- inability to trust; relationship difficulties

- alcohol and drug addiction

- eating disorders

Chapter 6

Elder Abuse

Elder mistreatment means that someone either does something, or fails to do something, that harms an elderly person or threatens the health and welfare of an elderly person.

Elder Mistreatment In The Family, Formal Care Settings, And The Community

Elder mistreatment can occur in many environments, including within the family, in formal care settings, or in the community or society at large.

The Family

Within the family, elder mistreatment is often seen in the context of care giving. For example, a caregiver may be overwhelmed or may not know what is needed or expected in providing care for the elderly person. Sometimes, a caregiver is reluctant to take on the role. Elder mistreatment can also be seen in the family when someone dependent on the older person reacts inappropriately to the older person's increasing frailty. An example of this situation might be when an adult child with mental illness reacts with anger or anxiety to a parent's decreased ability to provide care.

Formal Care Settings

Within formal care settings, when elder mistreatment occurs, it is attributable to those on staff who provide direct patient care (i.e., are in close contact with patients) but who have not had adequate training.

The Community

Within the community or society at large, the elderly are all too often subject to mistreatment by unscrupulous business people or other criminals.

Forms Of Elder Mistreatment

Elder mistreatment can take a number of different forms, including the following:

- Physical abuse

- Emotional abuse

- Neglect (intentional or unintentional)

- Financial exploitation

- Abandonment

- A combination of these

> ♣ **It's A Fact!!**
> Research suggests that 700,000 to 1.2 million elderly people (i.e., 4% of all adults older than 65) are subjected to elder mistreatment in the United States and that there are 450,000 new cases annually.

Risk Factors For Elder Mistreatment

Many factors can increase the risk of elder mistreatment.

Dependency Issues

- Dependency of the elderly person for care giving needs

- Dependency of another person on the elderly person

- Mental impairment in the dependent person or the caregiver (or both)

- Isolation of the dependent person or the caregiver (or both)

- Living arrangements inadequate for the needs of the dependent person

- Inability to perform daily functions

- Frailty

Family Issues

- Family conflict

- Family history of abusive behavior, alcohol or drug abuse, mental illness, or mental retardation

- Stressful family events, e.g., death of a loved one, loss of employment

Table 6.1. Visible Signs That Raise Suspicion Of Elder Mistreatment

Type of Mistreatment	Examples
Abandonment	Older person left alone frequently
Abuse	Many trips to the emergency room
	Fractures or bruises, some old and some new, especially bruises on both sides of inner arms and thighs
	Repeated falls
	Unexplained hair loss, possibly from pulling
Exploitation	Evidence that the victim's possessions are being taken by the caregiver
	Evidence that the victim's possessions (e.g., house, jewelry, car) are being taken over without their consent or approval
	Unexplained loss of social security or pension checks
	Dependent person's living conditions or appearance and his or her financial situation are inconsistent with each other
	Sudden inability to pay for food, health care, or other basic needs
	Unusual interest on the part of caregivers in the patient's assets
Neglect	Unexplained skin rashes, irritation, or ulcers
	Inappropriate dress
	No energy or spirit
	Malnourishment
	Poor hygiene (e.g., dirty, urine or fecal odor)
	Reports of being left in unsafe situation
	Reports of inability to get needed medication

Financial Issues

• Poverty

• Financial stress or lack of money for new health care needs

Institutional Concerns

• Socioeconomic factors within nursing homes, including poor working conditions, low salaries, inadequate staff training and supervision, prejudiced attitudes

Frail or debilitated older people may at times be incapable of helping themselves at all. In these situations, they many need more care than the caregiver is able to provide. In particular, mentally disturbed people who may behave in difficult ways (e.g., hitting, spitting, or screaming) can greatly add to the stress their caregiver feels, possibly causing the caregiver to respond with some form of elder mistreatment.

Clues To Possible Elder Mistreatment

Both visible signs and certain behaviors by either the elderly person or the caregiver can raise suspicion of elder mistreatment. Watching and talking to both the older person and their caregiver may provide clues that elder mistreatment may be happening. The behavior of victims of elder mistreatment in the presence of the person who might be abusing them may be significant.

Table 6.2. Behaviors That Raise Suspicion Of Elder Mistreatment

Possible Behaviors of the Victim	Possible Behaviors of the Caregiver(s)
Avoid eye contact or dart eyes often	May be nervous and fearful, or quiet and passive
Sit a distance away from caregiver	May try to prevent private conversation or examination of the elderly person
Cringe, back off, or startle easily as if expecting to be hit	Gives explanations of elderly person's injuries that don't make sense
Allow caregiver to answer for them all the time	May be impatient, irritable, and make negative or demeaning statements about the elderly person

---

Where To Go For Help   ✔ **Quick Tip**

If you think someone you know is a victim of elder mistreatment, you can ask
for help and advice from a number of resources:

- Your family doctor or another knowledgeable health professional
- Social workers, psychologists, or psychiatrists in your community
- Your state's Adult Protective Services (can provide relevant information
  and often direct assistance)
- The National Center on Elder Abuse (a good starting point in the search
  for information and resources); web link: http://elderabusecenter.org

---

Keeping A Perspective

It is important to remember that signs and symptoms that look like inadequate
or neglectful care giving may in fact be because of the dependent person's physical
or emotional disorders. For example, weight loss may be seen in a person with a
history of depression. In addition, in chronic progressive conditions, such as
Alzheimer's disease, deterioration is inevitable, even with the best of care.

It is also important to remember that the relationship of the elderly person with the caregiver(s) can be very complex, and the true cause of the
problem may not be obvious. In some cases, the elderly person is truly a
victim, while in others, the relationship between the elderly person and the
caregiver can be mutually abusive. There are even situations when the elderly person knowingly is part of the reason for the mistreatment. Of course,
there are many cases in which the older person and his or her caregivers are
making the best of a difficult and sometimes tragic situation.

What To Expect

When you suspect elder mistreatment and visit your doctor or other
health care provider, he or she will likely take a number of actions. First,
the situation is reported to Adult Protective Services and possibly other
public agencies (as required by your state). If the elderly person is in
immediate danger, your health care provider will make arrangements for
the person's safety. Possibilities are admitting the person to the hospital (if
needed for medical reasons), getting a court protective order, or making sure

the person is placed in a safe home. In all cases, the health care provider will make a complete evaluation of the person's physical, mental, and emotional status as well as the frequency, severity, and intent of the mistreatment.

If the suspicions of maltreatment are determined to be true, your health care provider will coordinate with Adult Protective Services in your state to find the option that least restricts the elderly person's independence.

If the elderly person is willing to accept voluntary services, he or she can receive several types including the following:

- Education about the tendency for elder mistreatment to happen more often and become more severe over time
- Safe home placement, court protective order, hospital admission
- Referral to drug or alcohol rehabilitation for the abuser(s) if appropriate
- Education, home health, or homemaker services for overburdened families and other caregivers
- Referral of the elderly person and family members for social work, counseling services, or legal assistance

If the elderly person is unwilling to accept voluntary services and has the capacity to make this decision, the health care provider will take the following actions:

- Educate the elderly person about the tendency for elder mistreatment to happen more often and become more severe over time
- Provide written information on emergency numbers and appropriate referrals
- Develop a follow-up plan

If the elderly person is unwilling to accept voluntary services and does not have the capacity to consent, the health care provider and Adult Protective Services will consider the following options:

- Financial management assistance
- Conservatorship
- Guardianship
- Committee
- Special court proceedings (e.g., orders of protection)

Chapter 7

Sexual Abuse

Sexual Assault Against Females

What is sexual assault?

Sexual assault is defined as any sort of sexual activity between two or more people in which one of the people is involved against his or her will.

The sexual activity involved in an assault can include many different experiences. Women can be the victims of unwanted touching, grabbing, oral sex, anal sex, sexual penetration with an object, and/or sexual intercourse.

There are a lot of ways that women can be involved in sexual activity against their will. The force used by the aggressor can be either physical or non-physical. Some women are forced or pressured into having sex with someone who has some form of authority over them (e.g., doctor, teacher, boss). Women can be bribed or manipulated into sexual activity against their will. Others may be unable to give their consent because they are under the influence of alcohol or drugs. In some cases, the sexual aggressor threatens to hurt the woman or people that she cares about. Finally, some assaults include physical force or violence.

About This Chapter: Information under the heading "Sexual Assault Against Females" is excerpted from "Sexual Assault against Females," by Sue Orsillo, Ph.D., National Center for Posttraumatic Stress Disorder, United States Department of Veterans Affairs, January 2007; "Men And Sexual Trauma" is excerpted from "Men and Sexual Trauma," by Julia M. Whealin, Ph.D., National Center for Posttraumatic Stress Disorder, January 2007.

Who commits sexual assaults?

Often, when we think about who commits sexual assault or rape, we imagine the aggressor is a stranger to the victim. Contrary to popular belief, sexual assault does not typically occur between strangers. The National Crime Victimization Survey, conducted by the U.S. Department of Justice, found that 76% of sexually assaulted women were attacked by a current or former husband, cohabitating partner, friend, or date. Strangers committed only 18% of the assaults that were reported in this survey.

How often do sexual assaults happen?

Estimating rates of sexual violence against women is a difficult task. Many factors stop women from reporting these crimes to police and to interviewers collecting statistics on the rate of crime in our country. Women may not want to report that they were assaulted because it is such a personal experience, because they blame themselves, because they are afraid of how others may react, and because they do not think it is useful to make such a report. However, there are statistics that demonstrate the magnitude of this problem in our country. For instance, a large-scale study conducted on several college campuses found that 20% of women reported that they had been raped in their lifetime. Another national study found that approximately 13–17% of women living in the U.S. have been the victims of completed rape, and an additional 14% of women were the victims of another form of sexual assault.

What happens to women after they are sexually assaulted?

After a sexual assault, women can experience a wide range of reactions. It is extremely important to note that there is no one pattern of response. Some women respond immediately, others may have delayed reactions. Some women are affected by the assault for a long time whereas others appear to recover rather quickly.

In the early stages, many women report feeling shock, confusion, anxiety, and/or numbness. Sometimes women will experience feelings of denial. In other words, they may not fully acknowledge what has happened to them, or they may downplay the intensity of the experience. This reaction may be more common among women who are assaulted by someone they know.

What are some early reactions to sexual assault?

In the first few days and weeks following the assault, it is very normal for a woman to experience intense and sometimes unpredictable emotions. She may have repeated strong memories of the event that are difficult to ignore, and nightmares are not uncommon. Women also report having difficulty concentrating and sleeping, and they may feel jumpy or on edge. While these initial reactions are normal and expected, some women may experience severe, highly disruptive symptoms that make it incredibly difficult to function in the first month following the assault. When these problems disrupt the woman's daily life, and prevent her from seeking assistance or telling friends and family members, the woman may have acute stress disorder (ASD). Symptoms of ASD include the following:

- feeling numb and detached, like being in a daze or a dream, or feeling that the world is strange and unreal

- difficulty remembering important parts of the assault

- reliving the assault through repeated thoughts, memories, or nightmares

- avoidance of things (places, thoughts, feelings) that remind the woman of the assault

- anxiety or increased arousal (e.g., difficulty sleeping, concentrating, etc.)

♣ It's A Fact!!

Studies estimate that one-third of women who are raped contemplate suicide, and 17% of rape victims actually attempt suicide.

Source: "Sexual Assault against Females," National Center for Posttraumatic Stress Disorder.

What are some other reactions that women have following a sexual assault?

Major Depressive Disorder (MDD): Depression is a common reaction following sexual assault. Symptoms of MDD can include a depressed mood, an inability to enjoy things, difficulty sleeping, changes in patterns of sleeping and eating, problems in concentration and decision-making, feelings of guilt, hopelessness, and decreased self-esteem. Research suggests that almost one-third of all rape victims have at least one period of MDD during their lives; and for many of these women, the depression can last for a long period of time. Thoughts about suicide are also common.

Anger: Many victims of sexual assault report struggling with anger after the assault. Although this is a natural reaction to such a violating event, there is some research that suggests that prolonged, intense anger can interfere with the recovery process and further disrupt a woman's life.

Shame And Guilt: These feelings are common reactions to sexual assault. Some women blame themselves for what has happened or feel shameful about being an assault victim. This reaction can be even stronger among women who are assaulted by someone that they know, or who do not receive support from their friends, family, or authorities, following the incident. Shame and guilt can also get in the way of a woman's recovery by preventing her from telling others about what happened and getting assistance.

Social Problems: Social problems can sometimes arise following a sexual assault. A woman can experience problems in her marital relationship or in her friendships. Sometimes an assault survivor will be too anxious or depressed to want to participate in social activities. Many women report difficulty trusting others after the assault, so it can be difficult to develop new relationships. Performance at work and school can also be affected.

Sexual Problems: Sexual problems can be among the most long-standing problems experienced by women who are the victims of sexual assault. Women can be afraid of, and try to avoid, any sexual activity. They may experience an overall decrease in sexual interest and desire.

Alcohol And Drug Use: Substance abuse can sometimes become problematic for women who are the victims of assault. A large-scale study found that compared to non-victims, rape survivors were 3.4 times more likely to use marijuana, 6 times more likely to use cocaine, and 10 times more likely to use other major drugs. Often, women will report that they use these substances to control other symptoms related to their assault.

Posttraumatic Stress Disorder (PTSD): Posttraumatic stress disorder (PTSD) involves a pattern of symptoms that some individuals develop after experiencing a traumatic event such as sexual assault. Symptoms of PTSD include repeated thoughts of the assault; memories and nightmares; avoidance of thoughts, feelings, and situations related to the assault; and increased arousal (e.g., difficulty sleeping and concentrating, jumpiness, irritability). One study that examined PTSD symptoms among women who were raped found that 94% of women experienced these symptoms during the two weeks immediately following the rape. Nine months later, about 30% of the women were still reporting this pattern of symptoms. The National Women's Study reported that almost one-third of all rape victims develop PTSD sometime during their lives, and 11% of rape victims currently suffer from the disorder.

Men And Sexual Trauma

At least 10% of men in our country have suffered from trauma as a result of sexual assault. Like women, men who experience sexual assault may suffer from depression, PTSD, and other emotional problems as a result. However, because men and women have different life experiences due to their different gender roles, emotional symptoms following trauma can look different in men than they do in women.

Who are the perpetrators of male sexual assault?

Those who sexually assault men or boys differ in a number of ways from those who assault only females.

Those who sexually assault males usually choose young men and male adolescents (the average age is 17 years old) as their victims and are more likely to assault many victims, compared to those who sexually assault females.

Perpetrators often assault young males in isolated areas where help is not readily available. For instance, a perpetrator who assaults males may pick up a teenage hitchhiker on a remote road or find some other way to isolate his intended victim.

As is true about those who assault and sexually abuse women and girls, most perpetrators of males are men. Specifically, men are perpetrators in about 86% of male victimization cases.

Despite popular belief that only gay men would sexually assault men or boys, most male perpetrators identify themselves as heterosexuals and often have consensual sexual relationships with women.

> ♣ **It's A Fact!!**
> Boys are more likely than girls to be sexually abused by strangers or by authority figures in organizations such as schools, the church, or athletics programs.
>
> Source: "Men and Sexual Trauma," National Center for Posttraumatic Stress Disorder.

What are some symptoms related to sexual trauma in boys and men?

Particularly when the assailant is a woman, the impact of sexual assault upon men may be downplayed by professionals and the public. However, men who have early sexual experiences with adults report problems in various areas at a much higher rate than those who do not.

Emotional Disorders: Men and boys who have been sexually assaulted are more likely to suffer from PTSD, other anxiety disorders, and depression than those who have never been abused sexually.

Substance Abuse: Men who have been sexually assaulted have a high incidence of alcohol and drug use. For example, the probability for alcohol problems in adulthood is about 80% for men who have experienced sexual abuse, as compared to 11% for men who have never been sexually abused.

Encopresis: One study revealed that a percentage of boys who suffer from encopresis (bowel incontinence) had been sexually abused.

Risk Taking Behavior: Exposure to sexual trauma can lead to risk-taking behavior during adolescence such as running away and other delinquent behaviors. Having been sexually assaulted also makes boys more likely to engage in behaviors that put them at risk for contracting HIV (such as having sex without using condoms).

How does male gender socialization affect the recognition of male sexual assault?

Men who have not dealt with the symptoms of their sexual assault may experience confusion about their sexuality and role as men (their gender role). This confusion occurs for many reasons. The traditional gender role for men in our society dictates that males be strong, self-reliant, and in control. Our society often does not recognize that men and boys can also be victims. Boys and men may be taught that being victimized implies that they are weak and, thus, not a man.

Furthermore, when the perpetrator of a sexual assault is a man, feelings of shame, stigmatization, and negative reactions from others may also result from the social taboos.

When the perpetrator of a sexual assault is a woman, some people do not take the assault seriously, and men may feel as though they are unheard and unrecognized as victims.

Parents often know very little about male sexual assault and may harm their male children who are sexually abused by downplaying or denying the experience.

What impact does gender socialization have upon men who have been sexually assaulted?

Because of their experience of sexual assault, some men attempt to prove their masculinity by becoming hyper-masculine. For example, some men deal with their experience of sexual assault by having multiple female sexual partners or engaging in dangerous "macho" behaviors to prove their masculinity. Parents of boys who have been sexually abused may inadvertently encourage this process.

Men who acknowledge their assault may have to struggle with feeling ignored and invalidated by others who do not recognize that men can also be victimized.

Because of these various gender-related issues, men are more likely than women to feel ashamed of the assault, to not talk about it, and to not seek help from professionals.

Are men who were sexually assaulted as children more likely to become child molesters?

Another myth that male victims of sexual assault face is the assumption that they will become abusers themselves. For instance, they may have heard that survivors of sexual abuse tend to repeat the cycle of abuse by abusing children themselves. Some research has shown that men who were sexually abused by men during their childhood have a greater number of sexual thoughts and fantasies about sexual contact with male children and adolescents. However, it is important to know that most male victims of child sexual abuse do not become sex offenders.

> ♣ **It's A Fact!!**
> Because of ignorance and myths about sexual abuse, men sometimes fear that the sexual assault by another man will cause them to become gay. This belief is false. Sexual assault does not cause someone to have a particular sexual orientation.
>
> Source: "Men and Sexual Trauma," National Center for Posttraumatic Stress Disorder.

Furthermore, many male perpetrators do not have a history of child sexual abuse. Rather, sexual offenders more often grew up in families where they suffered from several other forms of abuse such as physical and emotional. Men who assault others also have difficulty with empathy and thus put their own needs above the needs of their victims.

Is there help for men who have been sexually assaulted?

It is important for men who have been sexually assaulted to understand the connection between sexual assault and hyper-masculine, aggressive, and self-destructive behavior. Through therapy, men often learn to resist myths about what a "real man" is and adopt a more realistic model for safe and rewarding living.

It is important for men who have been sexually assaulted and who are confused about their sexual orientation to confront misleading societal ideas about sexual assault and homosexuality.

✔ Quick Tip

How To Protect Yourself From Being Sexually Assaulted

There are things you can do to reduce your chances of being sexually assaulted. Follow these tips from the National Crime Prevention Council:

- Be aware of your surroundings—who's out there and what's going on.

- Walk with confidence. The more confident you look, the stronger you appear.

- Do not let drugs or alcohol cloud your judgment.

- Be assertive—do not let anyone violate your space.

- Trust your instincts. If you feel uncomfortable in your surroundings, leave.

- Do not prop open self-locking doors.

- Lock your door and your windows, even if you leave for just a few minutes.

- Watch your keys. Do not lend them. Do not leave them. Do not lose them. And do not put your name and address on the key ring.

- Watch out for unwanted visitors. Know who's on the other side of the door before you open it.

- Be wary of isolated spots, like underground garages, offices after business hours, and apartment laundry rooms.

- Avoid walking or jogging alone, especially at night. Vary your route. Stay in well-traveled, well-lit areas.

- Have your key ready to use before you reach the door—home, car, or work.

- Park in well-lit areas and lock the car, even if you will only be gone a few minutes.

- Drive on well-traveled streets, with doors and windows locked.

- Never hitchhike or pick up a hitchhiker.

- Keep your car in good shape with plenty of gas in the tank.

- In case of car trouble, call for help on your cellular phone. If you do not have a phone, put the hood up, lock the doors, and put a banner in the rear mirror that says, "Help. Call police."

Source: Excerpted from "Sexual Assault," The National Women's Health Information Center, U.S. Department of Health and Human Services, Office On Women's Health, January 2005.

Men who have been assaulted often feel stigmatized, which can be the most damaging aspect of the assault. It is important for men to discuss the assault with a caring and unbiased support person, whether that person is a friend, clergyman, or clinician. However, it is vital that this person be knowledgeable about sexual assault and men.

A local rape crisis center may be able to refer men to mental health practitioners who are well informed about the needs of male sexual assault victims.

Chapter 8

Incest

Introduction

Incest is often included as a subset of sexual assault of children. While there is a substantial amount of overlap in the two types of assault, for the purposes of this chapter, we have separated them in recognition of the different needs that victims of each type of assault may have.

Definition

Sexual contact between persons who are so closely related that their marriage is illegal (e.g., parents and children, uncles/aunts and nieces/nephews, etc.). This usually takes the form of an older family member sexually abusing a child or adolescent.

Incest is considered by many experts to be a particularly damaging form of sexual abuse because it is perpetrated by individuals whom the victim trusts and depends upon. In addition, support can also be lacking and pressure to keep silent powerful, as fear of the family breaking up can be overwhelming to other family members.

There are, however, different cultural expectations and rules about incest. For instance, in some areas of the Arab world and southern India, it is

About This Chapter: Information in this chapter is from "Incest." © 2006 Rape, Abuse and Incest National Network (www.rainn.org). Reprinted with permission.

estimated that as many as 50% of marriages occur between first cousins. In addition, in southern India it is still common to see a maternal uncle (the mother's brother) marry the first daughter.

Incest can include such sexual acts as the following:

- non-contact acts—sexual comments, exposure, voyeurism, showing pornographic materials, etc.
- sexual contact—touching, rubbing
- digital or object penetration—both of the victim and of the perpetrator
- oral sex—both of the victim and of the perpetrator
- penile penetration—vaginal, anal, animals

Circumstances of the sexual acts can also be diverse including the following:

- dyadic sexual abuse—involving two people (victim and perpetrator)
- group sex
- sex rings
- sexual exploitation
- child pornography
- child prostitution

Common Reactions

Reactions In Children

- withdrawal
- depression
- sleeping and eating disorders
- self-mutilation
- phobias
- psychosomatic symptoms (stomach aches, headaches)
- school problems (absences, drops in grades)

- poor hygiene/excessive bathing

- anxiety

- guilt

- regressive behaviors— thumb sucking, etc.

Reactions In Children, Adolescents, And Adults

Traumatic Sexualization

- aversive feelings about sex

- overvaluing sex

- sexual identity problems

- hypersexual or sexual avoidance

Stigmatization

- feelings of guilt/responsibility for the abuse

- self-destructive behavior
  - substance abuse
  - self-harm
  - suicidal ideation
  - risk-taking acts
  - provocative behavior in order to incite punishment

✎ What's It Mean?

The exact definition of "rape," "sexual assault," "sexual abuse," and similar terms differs by state. The wording can get confusing, since states often use different words to mean the same thing, or use the same words to describe different things. For a precise legal definition, you need to check the law in your state. But here are some general guidelines based on the definitions used by the U.S. Justice Department. Please note that these definitions are somewhat graphic, which is inevitable when describing crimes this violent.

Rape: Rape is forced sexual intercourse, including vaginal, anal, or oral penetration. Penetration may be by a body part or an object. Rape victims may be forced through threats or physical means. In about 8 out of 10 rapes, no weapon is used other than physical force. Anyone may be a victim of rape: women, men, or children, straight or gay.

Sexual Assault: Sexual assault is unwanted sexual contact that stops short of rape or attempted rape. This includes sexual touching and fondling. (But, be aware: Some states use this term interchangeably with rape.)

Incest: Incest is sexual contact between persons who are so closely related that their marriage is illegal (e.g., parents and children, uncles/aunts and nieces/nephews, etc.). This usually takes the form of an older family member sexually abusing a child or adolescent.

Source: Excerpted from "What is Rape? What is Sexual Assault?" © 2006 Rape, Abuse and Incest National Network (www.rainn.org). Reprinted with permission.

Betrayal

- lack of trust, especially of those who were supposed to be protective and nurturing

- avoidance of investment in others

- manipulative behaviors

- anger, acting out, and borderline behaviors

- re-enacting the trauma through involvement in additional abusive or dangerous relationships

Powerlessness

- perception of vulnerability, victimization

- desire to control and prevail—often exhibited as identification with the aggressor

- avoidance—including dissociation, running away

- anxiety—including phobias, sleep problems, eating problems, elimination problems, revictimization

☞ **Remember!!**

It is important to note that there is no standard or typical symptom that can identify an individual as having survived incest. Much of the reactions and symptoms will depend on age at time of abuse, age at time of disclosure, support (or lack of support) from other caregivers, length of abuse, sex of the victim and perpetrator, etc.

Source: From "Incest." © 2006 Rape, Abuse and Incest National Network (www.rainn.org). Reprinted with permission.

Chapter 9

Stalking

Defining Stalking

Stalking creates uncertainty, instills fear, and can completely disrupt lives. It can involve severe, even lethal, violence. Stalking involves a pattern of overtly criminal and/or apparently innocent behavior that makes victims fear for themselves or others. Stalking is distinguishable from many other types of crime in two important ways. First, it entails repeat victimization of a person the offender targets; it is, by its very nature, a series of acts, rather than a single incident. Second, it is partly defined by its impact on the victim. While legal definitions of stalking vary from state to state, the following is a useful general definition: A course of conduct directed at a specific person that would cause a reasonable person fear.

Prevalence And Nature Of Stalking

Stalking is widespread. Nearly one in 12 women and one in 45 men are stalked at least once in their lifetime. It is estimated that more than a million women and nearly half a million men are stalked in the United States each year. The overwhelming majority (78 percent) of victims are women, and the majority of offenders (87 percent) are men.

About This Chapter: Information in this chapter is excerpted from *Stalking*, Office of Community Oriented Policing Services, U.S. Department of Justice, February 2006.

Most victims know their stalkers. Even though we often hear reports of fans stalking celebrities, survey evidence indicates that less than a quarter of female victims and a third of male victims are stalked by strangers. Nearly 60 percent of female victims and 30 percent of male victims are stalked by current or former intimate partners. In intimate partner cases, fewer than half of stalking incidents occur after the relationship ends. Most of the time, the stalking occurs during the relationship.

Stalking and domestic violence intersect in a variety of ways. Research indicates that 81 percent of women stalked by an intimate partner have been physically assaulted by that person. Thirty-one percent of women stalked by an intimate partner have been sexually assaulted by that person. Offenders who stalk former intimate partners are more likely to have physically or sexually assaulted them before the relationship ended.

Stalking is often a feature of relationships involving domestic violence. Like domestic violence, it is a crime of power and control. In one study about stalking and pre-stalking relationships, over 50 percent of the women were psychologically abused, 65 percent reported physical abuse, and 8.6 percent experienced sexual abuse during their relationship. If stalking is defined as a course of conduct that intimidates or frightens the victim, then relationships involving domestic violence also involve stalking.

Both domestic violence and stalking are linked to lethal violence. Research has revealed that one-third of women killed each year in the United States die at the hands of a current or former intimate. It is estimated that 25 to 35 percent of stalking cases involve violence; and when stalking leads to violence, it is often a precursor to lethal violence. Studies show that stalking precedes an exceedingly high proportion of homicides by intimates. In over 75 percent of completed and attempted female homicides by intimates, the offenders stalked the victims in the year before the offense.

♣ **It's A Fact!!**
In cases involving intimate partners, 21 percent of victims surveyed reported that stalking occurred during the relationship, 36 percent reported that it occurred both during and after the relationship, and 43 percent reported that it started after the relationship.

Victims report only about half of stalking incidents to the police. Generally, those who do not report do not think the matter is criminal, do not think the police can help them, or fear that reporting will make the stalker even more dangerous. Twenty percent of victims who reported stalking stated that the police did not act regarding their complaints. Other victims may not report incidents because they may minimize the risk a stalker poses or blame themselves for the stalker's behavior.

State And Federal Anti-Stalking Laws

The first stalking law was passed in California in 1990. Since then, increasing awareness about stalking's impact has led legislatures in all 50 states to pass stalking laws. While legislation is critical, laws alone accomplish little without clear anti-stalking policies and effective enforcement. Yet most police agencies across the country have not adopted distinct stalking-intervention protocols and procedures.

Stalking laws vary from state to state, but they share certain basic elements. Statutes generally define stalking in terms of a course of conduct or pattern of behavior that would cause a reasonable person to fear bodily injury or death for himself/herself or a member of his/her immediate family. Similarly, under most state laws, two or more incidents are required to establish a course of conduct. Because state laws vary, you should consult with your local prosecutor regarding your state's stalking law to be clear about what evidence is necessary to build a stalking case. In addition to specific stalking statutes, numerous other state and local laws relating to a wide variety of crimes and the investigation or prevention of crime may be relevant in stalking cases. These include laws governing the following:

- protective/restraining orders

- threats, assaults, and attempted murder

- kidnapping

- vandalism and other property crimes

- theft

- domestic violence

- sexual assault

- hate crimes

- terrorism or terrorist threats

- annoying phone calls and other forms
  of harassment

- identity theft

- utility theft

- wiretapping

✔ **Quick Tip**
You can find state stalking statutes on the National Center for Victims of Crime's Stalking Resource Center website, http://www.ncvc.org/src.

Federal statutes specifically relating to or applicable to stalking may provide further options for prosecuting stalkers.

Stalking Behaviors

Stalking, by definition, is not a one-time act but a course of conduct. It may involve a mix of patently criminal acts and acts that, in isolation, would seem non-threatening. It is the pattern and context of these criminal and non-criminal acts that constitute stalking.

Stalking often includes the following:

- assaulting the victim

- violating protective orders

- sexually assaulting the victim

- vandalizing the victim's property

- burglarizing the victim's home or otherwise stealing from the victim

- threatening the victim

- killing the victim's pet(s)

♣ **It's A Fact!!**
Sixty-nine percent of female and 81 percent of male victims with protective orders reported that their stalkers had violated the order.

Other common stalking behaviors include the following:

- sending the victim cards or gifts

- leaving telephone or e-mail messages for the victim

- disclosing to the victim personal information the offender has un-covered about him or her

- disseminating personal information about the victim to others

- following the victim

- visiting the victim at work

- waiting outside the victim's home

- sending the victim photographs taken of him or her without consent

- monitoring the victim's internet history and computer usage

- using technology to gather images of, or information about, the victim

Types Of Stalkers

While stalkers come from different backgrounds and have different per-sonalities, researchers have developed several widely accepted typologies of them. It is important to emphasize that, while stalker typologies can be helpful, they are only general classifications. Whenever possible, a properly trained professional should conduct a threat assessment. Individual stalkers may not precisely fit any single category and often exhibit characteristics associated with more than one category. However, the typology can alert investigators and victim advocates to certain general characteristics exhibited by similar stalkers and help them with threat assessment and safety planning.

One widely accepted typology of stalkers is based on the stalker's under-lying motives and includes the following categories:

- **Simple Obsessional:** This is the most common type. The stalker is usually a male and the victim an ex-spouse, ex-lover, or former boss. The stalking sometimes results from the stalker's feeling the victim has mistreated him or her. In intimate relationships, the stalking fre-quently begins before a breakup.

- **Love Obsessional:** The stalker is a stranger or casual acquaintance to the victim but is obsessed and begins a campaign of harassment to make the victim aware of his or her existence. This type often stalks a celebrity or public figure but can also stalk a non-celebrity.

- **Erotomania:** The stalker falsely believes that the victim is in love with him or her, and that, but for some external obstacle or interference, they would be together. The victim may be rich or famous or in a position of power (e.g., a movie star, employer, or political figure). In this situation, the stalker could also pose a great risk to those close to the victim (e.g., a spouse or lover perceived to be "in the way").

- **False Victimization Syndrome:** This is extremely rare and involves someone who consciously or subconsciously wants to play the role of victim. He or she may make up a complex tale claiming to be a stalking victim. In such cases, the would-be victim is sometimes the actual stalker and the alleged offender is the real victim.

Another typology used to classify stalkers identifies them by their relationship to the victim. This typology divides stalkers into two basic categories: intimate and non-intimate. The following is a brief description of these categories:

- **Intimate:** A former relationship exists between the stalker and the victim. There is likely a history of abuse, such as domestic violence, by the stalker. The stalker often seeks to reestablish a relationship the victim has tried to end.

- **Non-Intimate:** The stalker has no interpersonal relationship with the victim. He or she may choose the victim after a brief encounter or simply after observing the victim. The victim is often unable to identify the stalker when he or she first becomes aware of being stalked. This type is subdivided into the following two categories:

  - **Organized:** The relationship between the stalker and the victim is characterized by one-way, anonymous communication from stalker to victim. The stalker is methodical and calculating, and the victim usually does not know the stalker's identity.

- Delusional: The relationship between the stalker and the victim is based solely on the stalker's psychological fixation on the victim. The stalker is delusional and falsely believes he or she has a relationship or other connection with the victim.

Again, stalkers often exhibit behaviors from more than one typology.

Stalking's Impact On Victims

Unlike the case with many crimes, the legal definition of stalking covers not only the offender's behavior but also the effects on the victim. The victim's psychological responses and the changes the victim makes in his or her life as a result of stalking can all be used as evidence of the fear the offender has caused.

Stalking's impact is often wide-ranging, severe, and psychologically traumatic. Many victims feel constantly on alert, vulnerable, out of control, stressed, and anxious. Dealing with stalking can consume all their energy. They may experience a loss of trust, long-term emotional distress, and significant disruption of everyday living. Many seek psychological counseling. Victims' symptoms tend to worsen with each new incident and may be compounded by concerns about the effects on their children and other secondary victims.

♣ **It's A Fact!!**

Stalkers are, by their very nature, obsessive and dangerous. Regardless of typology, you should always consider stalkers capable of killing their victims. Anyone the stalker perceives as impeding his or her contact with the victim, including police, prosecutors, and advocates, is also at risk. Some stalkers seek union with their victims through murder-suicide. Any suicidal statements or gestures the stalker makes should serve as an indication that the stalker is a high-risk threat.

Stalking can also trigger a wide variety of behavioral reactions. Many victims take steps to avoid being followed and spied on. They alter their normal routines, avoid going out alone, and give up leisure activities. To protect themselves, they may screen all telephone calls (at home and work) and change their telephone number, e-mail and postal addresses, driver's license, and social security number. More drastic action may include temporary or permanent relocation.

They may move to another state or try to change their identity, often up-rooting children in the process, leaving behind close friends and relatives, and abandoning careers.

When the criminal justice system fails to protect victims from stalking, it makes it that much harder for them to recover from its effects.

Chapter 10

Sexual Harassment

What is sexual harassment?

Sexual harassment is a form of sex discrimination, which is a violation of Title VII of the Civil Rights Act of 1964. The Equal Employment Opportunity Commission (EEOC) guidelines define two types of sexual harassment: "quid pro quo" and "hostile environment."

What is "quid pro quo" sexual harassment?

Unwelcome sexual advances, requests for sexual favors, and other verbal or physical conduct of a sexual nature constitute "quid pro quo" sexual harassment when (1) submission to such conduct is made either explicitly or implicitly a term or condition of an individual's employment, or (2) submission to or rejection of such conduct by an individual is used as the basis for employment decisions affecting such an individual.

What is "hostile environment" sexual harassment?

Unwelcome sexual advances, requests for sexual favors, and other verbal or physical conduct of a sexual nature constitute "hostile environment" sexual

About This Chapter: Information in this chapter is from "Questions and Answers About Sexual Harassment," Food Safety and Inspection Service, United States Department of Agriculture, February 2006.

harassment when such conduct has the purpose or effect of unreasonably interfering with an individual's work performance or creating an intimidating, hostile, or offensive environment.

What factors determine whether an environment is hostile?

The central inquiry is whether the conduct "unreasonably interfered with an individual's work performance" or created "an intimidating, hostile, or offensive environment." The EEOC will look at the following factors to determine whether an environment is hostile: (1) whether the conduct was verbal, or physical, or both; (2) how frequently it was repeated; (3) whether the conduct was hostile or patently offensive; (4) whether the alleged harasser was a co-worker or supervisor; (5) whether others joined in perpetrating the harassment; and (6) whether the harassment was directed at more than one individual. No one factor controls. An assessment is made based upon the totality of the circumstances.

What is unwelcome sexual conduct?

Sexual conduct becomes unlawful only when it is unwelcome. The challenged conduct must be unwelcome in the sense that the person did not solicit or incite it, and in the sense that the person regarded the conduct as undesirable or offensive.

How will the EEOC determine whether conduct is unwelcome?

When confronted with conflicting evidence as to whether conduct was welcome, the EEOC will look at the record as a whole and at the totality of the circumstances, evaluating each situation on a case-by-case basis. The investigation should determine whether the victim's conduct was consistent, or inconsistent, with his/her assertion that the sexual conduct was unwelcome.

Who can be a victim of sexual harassment?

The victim may be a woman or a man. The victim does not have to be of the opposite sex. The victim does not have to be the person harassed but could be anyone affected by the offensive conduct.

Who can be a sexual harasser?

The harasser may be a woman or a man. He or she can be the victim's supervisor, an agent of the employer, a supervisor in another area, a co-worker, or a non-employee.

Can one incident constitute sexual harassment?

It depends. In "quid pro quo" cases, a single sexual advance may constitute harassment if it is linked to the granting or denial of employment or employment benefits. In contrast, unless the conduct is quite severe, a single incident or isolated incidents of offensive sexual conduct or remarks generally do not create a "hostile environment." A hostile environment claim usually requires a showing of a pattern of offensive conduct. However, a single, unusually severe incident of harassment may be sufficient to constitute a Title VII violation; the more severe the harassment, the less need to show a repetitive series of incidents. This is particularly true when the harassment is physical. For example, the EEOC will presume that the unwelcome, intentional touching of a charging party's intimate body areas is sufficiently offensive to alter the condition of his/her working environment and constitute a "hostile environment."

Can verbal remarks constitute sexual harassment?

Yes. The EEOC will evaluate the totality of the circumstances to ascertain the nature, frequency, context, and intended target of the remarks. Relevant factors may include (1) whether the remarks were hostile and derogatory; (2) whether the alleged harasser singled out the charging party; (3) whether the charging party participated in the exchange; and (4) the relationship between the charging party and the alleged harasser.

What should a sexual harassment victim do?

The victim should directly inform the harasser that the conduct is unwelcome and must stop. It is important for the victim to communicate that the conduct is unwelcome, particularly when the alleged harasser may have some reason to believe that the advance may be welcomed. However, a victim of harassment need not always confront his/her harasser directly, so long as his/her conduct demonstrates that the harasser's behavior is unwelcome. The victim should also use any employer complaint mechanism or grievance system available.

♣ It's A Fact!!
Sexual Harassment At School

Question: There is a boy at school who keeps touching my breasts like he's playing around. I don't think it's funny, and I want to know what to do.

Answer: What you describe here is a textbook example of schoolyard sexual harassment. Sexual harassment is any unwanted and/or inappropriate sexual touching and or language that makes the school environment feel unsafe and hostile. It is much more common than most people think.

While sexual harassment is well addressed on college and university campuses, it remains a taboo topic in high school and middle school settings. This is bad because much of our lifelong attitudes toward members of the opposite sex are formed in these early years. Unfortunately, a combination of outdated attitudes and stereotypes about uncontrollable teenage hormones keep the issue of sexual harassment at school from being discussed with any level of seriousness. It is much easier to take a "boys will be boys"; "it's all hormones, no brains"; or, "they haven't figured out the proper way to let a girl know they are interested" attitude than it is to admit that teens are capable of using sexually charged conduct as a weapon against others. It is easier to ignore the reality behind this type of behavior, and want to dismiss it as social bumbling, than it is to face reality. The irony is those teens that engage in this form of harassment do not need excuses made for them, they need to be held accountable.

While I doubt that this boy's intentions are to threaten or intimidate you, his actions are totally out of line. He needs to be shown and told that he has crossed a line with you. Next time this happens, firmly push his hand away and say, "I don't like it when you do that, I don't find it flattering, please stop!" If he becomes hostile, simply add, "I'm sorry you can't see my side of this and appreciate my feelings", and then walk away. Walk away and straight to the teacher or counselor that you trust most.

Since retaliation or hurtful rumors are always a fear with teens, I suggest a non-aggressive approach. Go to the teacher or counselor and tell them what has happened, tell them how often it has happened in the past, and that you were not sure how to handle it, so you kept quiet. Say that it became unbearable and you decided to say something to him. Tell the teacher what you said to stop him and how he reacted. Then say that since you are afraid he may get hostile, you would prefer that they not discipline him unless he refuses to stop despite your warning. Tell them that now that you have made your feelings known to him, that if the behavior continues, you will expect the school to get involved and discipline him; but for now, request that they just keep an extra eye on him. I also suggest repeating all of the above to your parents so that they can become involved if the behavior persists. If this boy keeps doing it, do not hesitate to insist that the school do something about it. They have a legal obligation to keep you safe and comfortable at school.

That said, if this boy acts this way towards other girls as well, we are not dealing with an inept teenage boy, we are dealing with a budding predator. If this is the case, he is using the sexual touching as a "social weapon" designed to intimidate and upset girls. He must be stopped with a firm hand and school intervention. If he is indeed doing this to cause others discomfort, the school should be alerted immediately. It is good if you can get together a group of his victims before going to the school; there is strength in numbers. Together you can all demand that he be reprimanded without fear that retaliatory gossip will discredit you. If this boy intimidates girls in this manner, he has a serious problem and needs professional help as soon as possible.

You are in the thick of it and are able to make a judgment call as to his motivations. If the boy has a crush on you, tell him that there are much better ways to get your attention and that him grabbing you the way he does only makes you less interested in being around him. Tell him if he wants to earn your affections, he can do it by being polite, courteous, and caring of your feelings. Then decide if you could ever be with him romantically and be honest with him about how you feel. However, if he is just a big pain who enjoys bugging girls in this manner, get the school involved and never bother with him again.

Chapter 11

Child Pornography

Defining Child Pornography

Legal Definitions

The idea of protecting children from sexual exploitation is relatively modern. As late as the 1880s in the United States, the age of consent for girls was just 10 years. In 1977, only two states had legislation specifically outlawing the use of children in obscene material. The first federal law concerning child pornography was passed in 1978, and the first laws that specifically referred to computers and child pornography were passed in 1988. Since that time, there has been a steady tightening of child pornography laws.

The following summarizes the current federal legal situation in the United States:

- A child is defined as any person under the age of 18. Legislation has attempted to broaden the law to include computer-generated images (virtual images that do not involve real children) and people over 18 who appear to be minors. However, the court overturned both of these provisions. Congress has subsequently made a number of amendments to tighten federal law in these areas.

About This Chapter: Information in this chapter is excerpted from *Child Pornography on the Internet*, Office of Community Oriented Policing Services, U.S. Department of Justice, May 2006.

- A different and more stringent standard is applied to images involving children than to images involving adults. Pornography involving a child does not have to involve obscene behavior but may include sexually explicit conduct that is lascivious or suggestive. For example, in United States v. Knox (1993), a man was convicted for possessing videos in which the camera focused on the clothed genital region of young girls.

- Possession of (not just production and trading of) child pornography is an offense. In the case of the internet, images do not have to be saved for an offense to have occurred—they simply need to have been accessed.

Most states have followed the federal lead with specific legislation, allowing state police to join federal agencies in the fight against child pornography. However, the exact nature of the legislation varies considerably among states. There is also a wide variation in international laws covering child pornography, and this can have significant implications for law enforcement.

Non-Legal Definitions

Because legal definitions of both child and pornography differ considerably among jurisdictions, for research purposes child pornography is often defined broadly as any record of sexual activity involving a prepubescent person. Pornographic records include still photographs, videos, and audio recordings. The images themselves vary considerably in their graphic content. In some cases, individuals may collect images that do not involve overt pornography and are not technically illegal. There are ten levels of image severity, and they are as follows:

1. **Indicative:** Non-sexualized pictures collected from legitimate sources (e.g., magazines, catalogs).

2. **Nudist:** Naked or semi-naked pictures of children in appropriate settings collected from legitimate sources.

3. **Erotica:** Pictures taken secretly of children in which they reveal varying degrees of nakedness.

4. **Posing:** Posed pictures of children in varying degrees of nakedness.

5. **Erotic Posing:** Pictures of children in sexualized poses and in varying degrees of nakedness.

6. **Explicit Erotic Posing:** Pictures emphasizing the genitals.

7. **Explicit Sexual Activity:** Record of sexual activity involving children but not involving adults.

8. **Assault:** Record of children subjected to sexual abuse involving digital touching with adults.

9. **Gross Assault:** Record of children subjected to sexual abuse involving penetrative sex, masturbation, or oral sex with adults.

10. **Sadistic/Bestiality:** Record of children subjected to pain or engaging in sexual activity with an animal.

The Role Of The Internet In Promoting Child Pornography

The internet has escalated the problem of child pornography by increasing the amount of material available, the efficiency of its distribution, and the ease of its accessibility. Specifically, the internet does the following:

- permits access to vast quantities of pornographic images from around the world

- makes pornography instantly available at any time or place

- allows pornography to be accessed (apparently) anonymously and privately

- facilitates direct communication and image sharing among users

- delivers pornography relatively inexpensively

- provides images that are of high digital quality, do not deteriorate, and can be conveniently stored

- provides for a variety of formats (pictures, videos, sound), as well as the potential for real-time and interactive experiences

- permits access to digital images that have been modified to create composite or virtual images (morphing)

Components Of The Problem

The problem of internet child pornography can be divided into three components—the production, distribution, and downloading of images. In some cases, the same people are involved in each stage. However, some producers and/or distributors of child pornography are motivated solely by financial gain and are not themselves sexually attracted to children.

Production

This involves the creation of pornographic images. Collectors place a premium on new child pornography material. However, many images circulating on the internet may be decades old, taken from earlier magazines and films. Images may be produced professionally, and in these cases, often document the abuse of children in third-world countries. However, more commonly, amateurs make records of their own sexual abuse exploits, particularly now that electronic recording devices such as digital cameras and web cams permit individuals to create high quality, homemade images.

♣ **It's A Fact!!**
With the advent of multimedia messaging (MMR) mobile phones, clandestine photography of children in public areas is becoming an increasing problem.

Distribution

This involves the uploading and dissemination of pornographic images. These images may be stored on servers located almost anywhere in the world. Distribution may involve sophisticated pedophile rings or organized crime groups that operate for profit; but in many cases, is carried out by individual amateurs who seek no financial reward. Child pornography may be uploaded to the internet on websites or exchanged via e-mail, instant messages, newsgroups, bulletin boards, chat rooms, and peer-to-peer (P2P) networks. Efforts by law enforcement agencies and internet service providers (ISPs) to stop the dissemination of child pornography on the internet have led to changes in offenders' methods. Child pornography websites are often shut down as soon as they are discovered, and openly trading in pornography via e-mail or chat rooms is risky because of the possibility of becoming ensnared in a police sting operation (e.g., undercover police entering chat rooms posing as pedophiles or as minor children). Increasingly, those distributing child pornography are employing more sophisticated security measures to elude detection and are being driven to hidden levels of the internet.

Downloading

This involves accessing child pornography via the internet. The images do not need to be saved to the computer's hard drive or to a removable disk to constitute downloading. In some cases a person may receive spam advertising child pornography, a pop-up link may appear in unrelated websites, or he may inadvertently go to a child pornography website (e.g., by mistyping a key word). In most cases, however, users must actively seek out pornographic websites or subscribe to a group dedicated to child pornography. In fact, it has been argued that genuine child pornography is relatively rare in open areas of the internet, and increasingly, those seeking to find images need good computer skills and inside knowledge of where to look. Most child pornography is downloaded via newsgroups and chat rooms. Access to websites and online pedophile groups may be closed and require paying a fee or using a password.

Extent Of The Problem

It is difficult to be precise about the extent of internet child pornography, but all of the available evidence points to it being a major and growing problem. At any one time there are estimated to be more than one million pornographic images of children on the internet, with 200 new images posted daily. One offender arrested in the United Kingdom possessed 450,000 child pornography images. It has been reported that a single child pornography site received a million hits in a month. As noted above, one problem in estimating the number of sites is that many exist only for a brief period before they are shut down, and much of the trade in child pornography takes place at hidden levels of the internet.

> ♣ **It's A Fact!!**
> It has been estimated that there are between 50,000 and 100,000 pedophiles involved in organized pornography rings around the world, and that one-third of these operate from the United States.

Profile Of Users

There is no one type of internet child pornography user, and there is no easy way to recognize an offender. Having a preconceived idea of a child sex offender can be unhelpful and prove a distraction for investigating police. The following is true of users of internet child pornography:

- They are not necessarily involved in hands-on sexual abuse of children. It is not known exactly how many people may access child pornography on the internet without ever physically abusing a child. Before the internet, between one-fifth and one-third of people arrested for possession of child pornography were also involved in actual abuse. However, the internet makes it easy for people who may never have actively sought out traditional forms of child pornography to satisfy their curiosity online, and this may encourage casual users. Looking at the relationship from the other direction, those convicted of sexually abusing children will not necessarily seek out or collect child pornography, with one study putting the number of offenders who do so at around ten percent. The term child molester covers a wide variety of offenders, from serial predators to situational offenders who may not have ingrained sexual interest in children.

- They may come from all walks of life and show few warning signs. In fact, users of child pornography on the internet are more than likely to be in a relationship, to be employed, to have an above average IQ, to be college educated, and to not have a criminal record. Those arrested for online child pornography crimes have included judges, dentists, teachers, academics, rock stars, soldiers, and police officers.

A Psychological Typology

Sexual attraction to children is known as pedophilia. However, an interest in internet child pornography may be best thought of as falling along a continuum rather than in terms of a hard and fast

> ♣ **It's A Fact!!**
> Among the few distinguishing features of offenders are that they are likely to be white, male, and between the ages of 26 and 40, and may be heavy internet users to the extent that it interferes with other aspects of their lives.

distinction between pedophiles and non-pedophiles. People can behave very differently on the internet than they do in other areas of their lives. Interacting anonymously with a computer in the safety of one's own home encourages people to express hidden thoughts and desires. Offenders vary in the strength of their interest in child pornography, as well as in the level of severity of the pornographic image to which they are attracted. From a psychological perspective, based on a typology of general pornography users, the following categories of internet child pornography users are suggested:

1. **Recreational Users:** They access child pornography sites on impulse, out of curiosity, or for short-term entertainment. They are not seen to have long-term problems associated with child pornography use.

2. **At-Risk Users:** They are vulnerable individuals who have developed an interest in child pornography but may not have done so had it not been for the internet.

3. **Sexual Compulsives:** They have a specific interest in children as sexual objects and seek out child pornography.

An Offending Typology

Variations among offenders translate into different patterns of internet behavior. Offenders vary in the level of their involvement in internet child pornography, the degree of networking in which they engage with other offenders, their expertise in employing security strategies to avoid detection, and the extent to which their internet behavior involves direct sexual abuse of children. The following typology of child pornography offending has been suggested:

1. **Browsers:** Offenders who stumble across child pornography but knowingly save the images. They are not involved in networking with other offenders and do not employ security strategies to avoid detection. Their browsing is an indirect abuse of children.

2. **Private Fantasizers:** Offenders who create digital images (e.g., through morphing) for private use to satisfy personal sexual desires. These offenders do not network with other offenders, do not employ security strategies, and their private fantasies are an indirect abuse of victims.

3. **Trawlers:** Offenders who seek child pornography on the web through open browsers. They may engage in minimal networking, but they employ few security strategies and their trawling is an indirect abuse of victims.

4. **Non-Secure Collectors:** Offenders who seek child pornography in non-secure chat rooms (i.e., chat rooms that do not employ security barriers such as passwords) and other open levels of the internet. They are involved in relatively high levels of networking, and by definition, do not employ security strategies. Their collecting behavior is an indirect abuse of children. Because of the non-secured nature of their activities, there are limits to the number and nature of the images they can collect.

5. **Secure Collectors:** Offenders who are members of a closed newsgroup or other secret pedophile ring. They engage in high levels of networking and employ sophisticated security measures to protect their activities from detection. Their collecting behavior is an indirect abuse of children. Because they occupy hidden levels of the internet, they have access to a wide range of images. They may engage in obsessive levels of collecting, which not only involves amassing huge numbers of images, but also carefully cataloging and cross referencing them. As with other types of collections, they may expend considerable effort in obtaining rare and highly prized images. The collection may become an end in itself.

6. **Groomers:** Offenders who develop online relationships with children and send pornography to children as part of the grooming process. Grooming involves direct abuse of children. They may or may not be involved in wider networking with other offenders, but their contact with children exposes them to risk of detection. The child may tell someone about the relationship, or the offender may be unwittingly communicating with an undercover police officer.

7. **Physical Abusers:** Offenders who sexually abuse children and for whom an interest in child pornography is just part of their pedophilic interests. They may record their own abuse behaviors for their personal use, in which case, from a legal standpoint, the possession of pornography is secondary to the evidence of their abusive behavior that it records. They

may or may not network. By definition, a physical abuser directly abuses victims and his security depends upon the child's silence.

8. **Producers:** Offenders who record the sexual abuse of children for the purpose of disseminating it to others. The extent of their networking varies depending on whether they are also distributors. Again, the producer's direct abuse of the victim compromises his security.

9. **Distributors:** Offenders involved in disseminating abuse images. In some cases they have a purely financial interest in child pornography. More often, offenders at any of the above levels who share images may be classified as distributors. Thus, the extent of a distributor's networking, his level of security, and whether he engages in direct abuse of children depends upon the level at which he is operating.

♣ It's A Fact!!
Effects On The Children Portrayed

The vast majority of children who appear in child pornography have not been abducted or physically forced to participate. In most cases they know the producer—it may even be their father—and are manipulated into taking part by more subtle means. Nevertheless, to be the subject of child pornography can have devastating physical, social, and psychological effects on children.

The children portrayed in child pornography are first victimized when their abuse is perpetrated and recorded. They are further victimized each time that record is accessed. In one study, 100 victims of child pornography were interviewed about the effects of their exploitation—at the time it occurred and in later years. Referring to when the abuse was taking place, victims described the physical pain (e.g., around the genitals), accompanying somatic symptoms (such as headaches, loss of appetite, and sleeplessness), and feelings of psychological distress (emotional isolation, anxiety, and fear). However, most also felt a pressure to cooperate with the offender and not to disclose the offense, both out of loyalty to the offender and a sense of shame about their own behavior. Only five cases were ultimately reported to authorities. In later years, the victims reported that initial feelings of shame and anxiety did not fade but intensified to feelings of deep despair, worthlessness, and hopelessness. Their experience had provided them with a distorted model of sexuality, and many had particular difficulties in establishing and maintaining healthy emotional and sexual relationships.

Chapter 12

Commercial Child Sexual Exploitation: Sexual Activities For Money

Many trafficked children are destined for sex work, but many other children who have not been trafficked are also sexually abused for commercial gain. At least 97 countries have reported cases of the commercial sexual exploitation of children. It will always be difficult to say how many children are involved. This is a clandestine and criminal activity, and given their intense feeling of shame, most children never report the abuse. The last recorded estimates indicate that as many as two million children, mainly girls but also a significant number of boys, are sexually exploited in the multi-billion dollar commercial sex trade each year. At any time, therefore, several million children will be engaged in sex work. In Southeast Asia alone, it is thought that one million children are involved.

Children In The Sex Industry

Although many children are forced to enter the sex industry, others are driven to it out of economic necessity, attracted by the high incomes they can earn. In Viet Nam, for example, children working as prostitutes in central Hanoi can earn $1,000 per month, when the average monthly wage is $25.

About This Chapter: Information in this chapter is from "End Child Exploitation." Reproduced from the UNICEF UK website, www.unicef.org.uk, © UNICEF, January 2007.

The sex industry, for both adults and children, comes in many different forms, some organized, some more casual. At the more formal end of the spectrum, sex is specifically traded as a commodity—bought and sold through brothels and bars, for example, or in the form of pornographic images.

Children may also work independently, offering themselves for cash, as do many of the 10,000 to 15,000 boys selling themselves to sex tourists on the beaches of Sri Lanka.

♣ **It's A Fact!!**
Commercial sexual exploitation of children can be defined as "children, both male and female, engaging in sexual activities for money, profit, or any other consideration due to coercion or influence by any adult, syndicate, or group". The profit could go either to the child or to any third party involved in the transaction.

But the sex trade can also take on more indirect forms—looser arrangements where the children offer adults a range of services, some sexual, some not, in exchange for food or clothing, or shelter, or some kind of protection. There can also be relationships that are not overtly commercial, where adults—parents, teachers, priests, or youth workers—who have some authority over children, may also offer gifts to encourage them to keep quiet about abuse. The dividing lines between commercial and non-commercial exploitation are thus hard to draw. But at its heart, it is an exploitative relationship where adults use their superior power, physical or financial, to ensure that children comply with their sexual demands.

Working Conditions

Many of the children working in the sex industry do so in horrific conditions. This is especially true of children who have been trafficked, who may be effectively imprisoned in the brothels. Most children working in brothels do so under very difficult circumstances. In Cambodia, for example, one survey of 53 girls found that most lived in small dark rooms and served five to ten customers per day. Almost all had suffered physical abuse at the hands of brothel owners and customers, the most common forms being hitting and kicking. Children in brothels have also been drugged to make them submissive. On the other hand, they may have turned to prostitution to maintain a drug habit.

Children working in brothels are also exposed continually to a wide range of sexually transmitted infections (STIs), as well as early pregnancy and repeated abortions. But probably the greatest menace for child prostitutes nowadays is HIV/AIDS. A number of men now specifically seek out children for sex assuming that they are less likely to be infected. Some people who are HIV-positive even believe that sex with children, and particularly virgins, will remove their own infection. While many adult sex workers now insist that their clients use condoms, children are in a weaker position, either because they do not appreciate the danger, or because they are powerless to insist on condom use.

Beyond the health risk for children involved in sex work, there is also psychosocial damage, especially for children who have been trafficked. The violent and intimidating atmosphere engenders a feeling of isolation, helplessness, and lack of control—heightened by the fear of arrest. There is also social stigma. Children in Viet Nam, for example, say that one of their worries is that people from their home village will recognize them. All this can produce anxiety and depressive states including trauma.

♣ It's A Fact!!
Child Pornography

One of the most insidious and pervasive aspects of the commercial sexual exploitation of children is through the distribution of child pornography. In the past, this was distributed to a more limited extent through photographs and magazines. But the internet has opened up a plethora of new channels and drawn in many new users. Much of this material is generated as a record of sexual abuse by pedophiles and is often exchanged rather than sold. Nevertheless, such images are also available for sale on commercial sites. It also seems likely that organized crime is moving in. Since this is a clandestine activity, statistics are scarce, but the scale of the problem is evident from the result of just one operation. A child pornography ring that has since been broken up, the "Wonderland Club", had 180 known members spread across 49 countries, possessing 750,000 pornographic images and over 1,800 hours of digital video.

Child Sex Tourism

Most exploitation of children takes place as a result of their absorption into the adult sex trade where local people exploit them. In the Philippines, for example, it is thought that nine out of ten customers of child prostitutes are Filipinos. Nevertheless, the 1980s and 1990s have also seen an increase in tourism with a sexual component—sometimes deliberate "sex tourism" by pedophiles seeking out younger children, but more often by men or women who regard it as permissible to have sex with local people regardless of their age and who take the opportunity to exploit adolescents. While sex tourism is well established in many Asian countries, it is now emerging in other parts of the developing world, including West Africa.

Many of these adults do not consider themselves to be exploiters. They tell themselves that the children have actively chosen prostitution and have made the first approach, and that they come from cultures where children are naturally freer and more sexually experienced at an early age. They also argue that these children desperately need the money, so really they are doing them a favor. None of these rationalizations, however, can excuse a grievous abuse of power.

Chapter 13

Use Of Computers In The Sexual Exploitation Of Children

As more and more people discover the ability to communicate faster and more efficiently through computers and the internet, the possibility that predators will use these tools to advance their criminal activities also increases. The first online services were oriented toward adults, but children now make up one of the fastest growing populations of internet users. Nearly 30 million children and youth go online each year to research homework assignments, play games, and meet friends. This increased access to computer technology puts children at greater risk of sexual exploitation. Criminals involved in the sexual exploitation of children use the computer as a convenient tool to enter the homes of their victims, correspond with one another, and exchange images of illicit activities with child victims.

What is child sexual exploitation? As used in this chapter, the term "child sexual exploitation" refers to the sexual victimization of children and covers many different types of child sexual abuse. Child sexual exploitation encompasses more than physical sexual molestation. Any display or suggestion of sexual activity involving children, including written or graphic material, can be considered child sexual exploitation. Such material ranges from depictions of explicit sexual

About This Chapter: Information in this chapter is from *Use of Computers in the Sexual Exploitation of Children, Second Edition*, by Daniel S. Armagh and Nick L. Battaglia, Office of Juvenile Justice and Delinquency Prevention, Office of Justice Programs, U.S. Department of Justice, December 2006.

acts performed by children with adults, or children with children, to images depicting a fully dressed child in a sexual pose. The material need not meet the legal definition of child pornography. Nonsexual images of a child intermixed in a graphic display with other media that suggests sexually oriented activity can be considered child sexual exploitation.

♣ It's A Fact!!
Nineteen percent of children ages 10–17 surveyed in the U.S. Department of Justice's (DOJ's) Youth Internet Safety Survey received unwanted sexual solicitations online.

Cases of computer-facilitated child sexual exploitation may involve members of the child's own family (intrafamilial offenders), although this is not typical. Most child sexual exploitation investigations will involve one or more perpetrators victimizing several children over long periods of time. The victims will engage in explicit sexual activity, and the predators will document that activity in text and/or graphics on some type of media. The evidence will show that the perpetrator sought out the child specifically for sexual activity—that his actions were premeditated as opposed to being a "crime of opportunity."

Note: Women can also be child predators. In this chapter, for simplicity's sake, the male pronoun is used to refer to all sexual offenders who prey on children.

Understand The Behavior Of Child Predators

Child predators—sexual offenders who act on their sexual interest directed toward children—come from all economic and social backgrounds. Other terms used for these offenders include "pedophile" and "preferential sex offender." However, these terms have specific clinical definitions. This chapter uses the term "child predator" because it is a nonclinical term that anyone can testify to in court. Experience gained through hundreds of investigations and interviews shows that the behavior of child predators usually develops in four stages. They are as follows:

• **Awareness:** An individual first comes to realize that he has a sexual interest in children. This interest may manifest itself in several ways. Usually, the individual gathers as much information as possible on the subject in an attempt to understand his feelings. In this early stage, the internet provides access both to a variety of information sources—

newspaper articles, newscasts, and to online chats with other individuals who may have similar interests.

- **Fantasy:** The individual uses the research that he has collected as a source for sexual fantasizing and stimulation. Eventually, the fantasy becomes more fixated, with an emphasis on child pornography. An individual using a computer will exchange e-mail with others who share the same interests and save these messages and all other related material using some type of computer storage medium.

- **Stalking:** Fantasy is no longer enough, and the individual is now compelled to seek closeness to actual children. The child predator will loiter at athletic events, parks, playgrounds, school bus stops, and other locations where children are found and may seek positions of trust in order to have access to children. Hardcore child pornography plays an important role at this stage. An individual using a computer will progress from online chats with others with the same interests to chats with potential victims. He may send them photos of himself in sexual poses and request similar sexual photos in return.

- **Molestation:** The individual molests a child. The predator using a computer sets up a meeting with the child with whom he has been corresponding. Depending on the predator, the meeting may lead either to a seduction or to abduction of the child.

Know How Child Predators Use Computers

Like other child predators, those who use computers may be compelled to collect child pornography and child erotica, correspond with other predators, and ultimately, solicit a child for sexual activity. The computer is a powerful tool that offers child predators an easy, efficient, and anonymous means of achieving all of these goals within the confines of their home, workplace, local library, or any other location that offers them access to a computer.

Organizing Their Collections

A child predator who is also a collector may save everything that relates to children. Before computers were widely available, predators often recorded their exploits in diaries. Now they can use word processing software to write about their experiences. Where child predators once saved photos in albums, now they can store and organize all information they collect on their computer's hard drive or a removable storage device. This material may include chat room text, chat room user profiles, pictures chat room users have placed in their profiles, any internet correspondence with a child, and child pornography. Child predators can hide text, digital images, graphics files, and video files by using passwords and/or encryption techniques.

Corresponding With Other Predators

Child predators may seek validation by communicating with other adults who have similar interests. The internet enables these individuals to exchange information and share child pornography with less risk of identification or discovery. For predators in the awareness stage, the internet offers a means to research their interests anonymously from the privacy of their own home.

Finding Potential Victims

Previously, predators loitered in parks. Now they no longer need to seduce a child in person. Using the internet, a predator can enter children's chat rooms to develop relationships and ultimately, solicit a child. Curious children may also stray into adult chat rooms that advertise themselves as discussing adult/child sexual relationships where the children become vulnerable to sexual exploitation.

Child predators enter children's chat rooms by posing as someone friendly or interesting to a child. The type of chat room can vary from educational to one devoted to a specific interest such as sports, music, movies, or television programs. Chat room participants fill out a profile that other users can see, listing their name, hobbies, and interests. The predator will check profiles of users to look for victims. After carrying on a dialog with the parties in the chat room, the predator usually will invite a potential victim into a "private chat room" not accessible to anyone else. The predator can download all conversation from the private chat room to a computer storage medium. Once the predator downloads this conversation, he can use it for fantasizing, share it with other child predators, or use it to blackmail the victim into a personal meeting.

Part Two

Violence And The Teen Experience

Chapter 14

Risk Factors For Youth Violence: An Overview

Introduction To Risk Factors

The concepts of risk are integral to public health. A risk factor is anything that increases the probability that a person will suffer harm. In the context of this chapter, risk factors increase the probability that a young person will become violent. The public health approach to youth violence involves identifying risk factors, determining how they work, making the public aware of these findings, and designing programs to prevent or stop the violence.

Risk factors for violence are not static. Their predictive value changes depending on when they occur in a young person's development, in what social context, and under what circumstances. Risk factors may be found in the individual, the environment, or the individual's ability to respond to the demands or requirements of the environment. Some factors come into play

About This Chapter: This includes information from "Introduction to Risk and Protective Factors" and "Risk Factors in Adolescence" from Chapter 4 of *Youth Violence: A Report of the Surgeon General*, Office of the Surgeon General, U.S. Department of Health and Human Services, January 2001.

during childhood, whereas others do not appear until adolescence. Some involve the family, others the neighborhood, the school, or the peer group. Some become less important as a person matures, while others persist throughout the life span. To complicate the picture even further, some factors may constitute risks during one stage of development but not another. Finally, the factors that predict the onset of violence are not necessarily the same as those that predict the continuation or cessation of violence.

♣ It's A Fact!!

Do Sexually Abused Kids Become Abusers?

It is widely believed that boys who are victims of sexual abuse become abusers themselves. Studies of pedophiles suggest this often is the case, but new research shows that the risk may be smaller than previously thought.

Roughly one in ten male victims of child sex abuse in a United Kingdom study later went on to abuse children as adults, but the risk was far greater for sexually victimized children who came from severely dysfunctional families. Family history of violence, sexual abuse by a female, maternal neglect, and lack of supervision were all associated with a threefold-increased risk that the abused would become an abuser. The study is reported in the February 8, 2003 issue of *The Lancet*.

"The message here is that sexual victimization alone is not sufficient to suggest a boy is likely to grow up to become a sex offender," says study author and psychiatrist Arnon Bentovim. "But our study does show that abused boys who grow up in families where they are exposed to a great deal of violence or neglect are at particular risk."

Bentovim and colleagues from London's Institute of Child Health identified 224 adult male victims of child sexual abuse whose childhood medical and social service records were available for review. They then searched arrest and prosecution records to determine their later criminal activity. Most of the subjects were 20 years old or older when the study was conducted.

Twenty-six of the 224 sex abuse victims (12%) later committed sexual offenses, and in almost all cases their victims were also children. Abused children who came from families where violence was common were more than three times as likely to become abusers, as were those who experienced maternal neglect and sexual abuse by females.

Violence prevention and intervention efforts hinge on identifying risk factors and determining when in the course of development they emerge. To be effective, such efforts must be appropriate to a youth's stage of development. A program that is effective in childhood may be ineffective in adolescence and vice versa. Moreover, the risk factors targeted by violence prevention programs may be different from those targeted by intervention programs, which are designed to prevent the reoccurrence of violence.

One-third of the adult abusers had been cruel to animals as children, compared with just 5% of the child abuse victims who did not grow up to commit sexual crimes; but abusers and non-abusers experienced similar levels of physical abuse as children, and there were few significant differences in the severity or characteristics of the sexual abuse they suffered.

"It is clear that prevention of sexual abuse involves not just treating the victim, but ensuring that the family environment is safe," Bentovim says. "If you leave a child in a family situation where he continues to be subjected to abuse, even if it is not sexual, you are probably wasting your time."

Child health specialist, Paul Bouvier, MD, says that the real incidence of abused boys becoming pedophiles themselves is probably higher than the United Kingdom study suggests because it only included sexual predators who had been caught.

In an editorial accompanying the study, Bouvier argues that much can be learned by studying child sexual abuse victims who do not go on to become sexual predators or experience long-lasting trauma.

"It is quite important to know the risks for these children to have a bad outcome," he says. "But it is also important to look at those who are resilient and who don't become abusers later in life. What are the characteristics of those who evolve beyond this experience and go on to have a meaningful life?"

Source: "Do Sexually Abused Kids Become Abusers?" by Salynn Boyles, Copyright 2003 by WebMD. Reproduced with permission of WebMD via the Copyright Clearance Center.

Risk factors are not necessarily causes. Researchers identify risk factors for youth violence by tracking the development of children and adolescents over the first two decades of life and measuring how frequently particular personal characteristics and social conditions at a given age are linked to violence at later stages of the life course.

As used in this chapter, risk factors are personal characteristics or environmental conditions that predict the onset, continuity, or escalation of violence.

Most of the risk factors identified do not appear to have a strong biological basis. Instead, it is theorized, they result from social learning or the combination of social learning and biological processes. This means that violent youths who have violent parents are far more likely to have modeled their behavior on their parents' behavior—to have learned violent behavior from them—than simply to have inherited it from them. Likewise, society's differing expectations of boys and girls—expecting boys to be more aggressive, for example—can result in learned behaviors that increase or decrease the risk of violence.

The bulk of the research that has been done on risk factors identifies and measures their predictive value separately, without taking into account the influence of other risk factors. More important than any individual factor, however, is the accumulation of risk factors. Risk factors usually exist in clusters, not in isolation. Children who are abused or neglected, for example, tend to be in poor families with single parents living in disadvantaged neighborhoods beset with violence, drug use, and crime. Studies of multiple risk factors have found that they have independent, additive effects; that is, the more risk factors a child is exposed to, the greater the likelihood that he or she will become violent. One study, for example, has found that a 10-year-old exposed to six or more risk factors is ten times as likely to be violent by age 18 as a 10-year-old exposed to only one factor.

❖ **It's A Fact!!**
Good relationships with parents during childhood will help in a successful transition to adolescence, but they do not guarantee it.

Source: Office of the Surgeon General, U.S. Department of Health and Human Services, January 2001.

Risk Factors In Adolescence

Violence increases dramatically in the second decade of life, peaking during late adolescence at 12 to 20 percent of all young people and dropping off again sharply by the early twenties. Some of these youths followed the childhood-onset trajectory, becoming violent before puberty and escalating their rate of offending during adolescence; but over half of all violent youths begin their violent behavior in mid- to late adolescence. These youths gave little indication of problem behavior in childhood and did not have poor relations with their parents.

There are numerous theories about why violence begins in adolescence, but a few themes run through most of them. Developmentally, puberty is accompanied by major physical and emotional changes that alter a young person's relationships and patterns of interaction with others. The transition into adolescence begins the move toward independence from parents and the need to establish one's own values, personal and sexual identity, and the skills and competencies needed to compete in adult society. Independence requires young people to renegotiate family rules and degree of supervision by parents, a process that can generate conflict and withdrawal from parents. At the same time, social networks expand, and relationships with peers and adults in new social contexts equal or exceed in importance the relationships with parents. The criteria for success and acceptance among peers and adults change.

Adapting to all of these changes in relationships, social contexts, status, and performance criteria can generate great stress, feelings of rejection, and anger at perceived or real failure. Young people may be attracted to violent behavior as a way of asserting their independence of the adult world and its rules, as a way of gaining the attention and respect of peers, as a way of compensating for limited personal competencies, or as a response to restricted opportunities for success at school or in the community.

Adolescents exposed to violence at home may experience some of the same emotions and difficulties as younger school-age children—for example, fear, guilt, anxiety, depression, and trouble concentrating in school. In addition, adolescents may feel more vulnerable to violence from peers at school or gangs in their neighborhood and hopeless about their lives and their odds of surviving

to adulthood. These young people may not experience the growing feelings of competence
that are important at their stage of development. Ultimately, their exposure to violence may lead them to become violent
themselves.

Risk Factors By Domain

Not surprisingly, different risk factors for violence assume importance in
adolescence. Family factors lose predictive value relative to peer-oriented risk factors such as weak social ties to conventional
peers, antisocial or delinquent friends, and
membership in a gang. Even involvement in gen-
eral offenses, which had the largest effect size in childhood, has only a moderate effect size in adolescence.

♣ It's A Fact!!
Studies have shown that
adolescents exposed to violence
are more likely to engage in violent acts, often as preemptive
strikes in the face of a perceived
threat.

Source: Office of the Surgeon
General, U.S. Department of
Health and Human Ser-
vices, January 2001.

Individual: In early adolescence, involvement in general offenses—that
is, illegal but not necessarily violent acts, including felonies—becomes a
moderate risk factor for violence between the ages of 15 and 18. Its predictive power lessens from childhood, largely because teenagers are somewhat
more likely than children to engage in illegal behavior.

Psychological conditions, notably restlessness, difficulty concentrating,
and risk taking, have small effect sizes in adolescence. Restlessness and difficulty concentrating can affect performance in school, a risk factor whose
importance increases slightly in adolescence. Risk taking gains predictive
power in early adolescence, particularly in combination with other factors. A
reckless youth who sees violence as an acceptable means of expression, for
example, is more likely to engage in violent behavior.

Aggressiveness exerts a small effect on later violence among adolescent
males, as does simply being male. While aggressiveness is unusual in children between the ages of about 6 and 10, it is not terribly unusual in adolescence. Similarly, physical violence and crimes against persons in early adolescence have a small effect on the likelihood of violence at ages 15 to 18.

Antisocial attitudes and beliefs, including hostility toward police and a positive attitude toward violence, are more important predictors among adolescent boys than they are among children, but their effect sizes remain small. Antisocial behavior and low IQ continue to have small effect sizes in adolescence.

Substance use, which was a strong predictor of later violence for children, poses a small risk of later violence for adolescents. The question as to whether drug use causes young people to become violent is complex and has been widely studied, but there is little compelling pharmacological evidence linking illicit drug use and violence. In one large study, youths reported that over 80 percent of the violent incidents they initiated had not been preceded by drug use including alcohol use. Thus, the risk may lie more in the characteristics of the social settings in which drug use and violence are likely to occur than in any effect of drugs on behavior.

The majority of violent adolescent offenders use alcohol and illicit drugs. Illicit drug use tends to begin after the onset of violence and to be associated with more frequent violent behavior and a longer criminal career. This finding suggests that drug use may contribute to continued violence rather than to the onset of violence, but it is far from conclusive. Evidence shows that some violent behavior stems from robberies or other attempts to get money to support a drug habit, but also that this link is relatively rare. If any substance can be said to cause youth violence, that substance is alcohol; however, this causal link is inconclusive because adolescent drinking is dependent to a large degree on the situation and social context in which it takes place.

Family: Parents' direct influence on behavior is largely eclipsed by peer influence during adolescence. Not surprisingly, therefore, most family risk factors diminish in importance, including the influence of antisocial parents and low socioeconomic status, the most powerful early risk factors. There are no large or even moderate risk factors in the family domain in adolescence.

Poor parent-child relations continue to have a small effect size, but for adolescents this category includes inadequate supervision and monitoring of young people's activities and low parental involvement, in addition to inappropriate discipline. Broken homes and parental abuse also exert small effects. Other adverse family conditions present a risk factor; for example, some studies have found that family conflict is a risk factor for violence among adolescent males.

Although parents can and do influence their adolescents' behavior, they do so largely indirectly. The kind of peers chosen by young people, for example, is related to the relationship they have with their parents.

School: There are no large or moderate risk factors for violence in the school domain, but poor attitude toward, or performance in school—particularly if it leads to academic failure—is a slightly larger risk factor in early adolescence than in childhood.

Research on school violence indicates that a culture of violence has arisen in some schools, adversely affecting not just students, but teachers and administrators as well. Students exposed to violence at school may react by staying home to avoid the threat or by taking weapons to school in order to defend themselves. For their part, teachers may burn out after years of dealing with discipline problems and threats of violence.

Schools located in socially disorganized neighborhoods are more likely to have a high rate of violence than schools in other neighborhoods. At the same time, however, researchers emphasize that most of the violence to which young people are exposed takes place in their home neighborhood, or the neighborhood surrounding the school, not in the school itself. Individual schools, like individual students, do not necessarily reflect the characteristics of the surrounding neighborhood. A stable, well-administered school in a violent neighborhood may function as a safe haven for students.

♣ It's A Fact!!

The chances of becoming a victim of violence are more than two and one-half times as great in schools where gangs are reported, and these schools are disproportionately located in disadvantaged, disorganized neighborhoods.

Source: Office of the Surgeon General, U.S. Department of Health and Human Services, January 2001.

Some gang activity takes place in schools, but school gangs are generally younger and less violent than street gangs, which form in neighborhoods. Gangs in schools increased dramatically (by 87 percent) between 1989 and 1995 but have recently declined.

Peer groups complicate the picture further. They operate both in neighborhoods and in schools, but the concentration of young people in schools may intensify the influence of these groups. One large study of adolescent males found that some schools have dominant peer groups that value academic achievement and disapprove of violence, while others have groups that approve of the use of violence. This study found that the risk of becoming involved in violence varied depending on the dominant peer culture in their school, regardless of their own views about the use of violence.

Peer Group: Peer groups are all-important in adolescence. Adolescents who have weak social ties—that is, who are not involved in conventional social activities and are unpopular at school—are at high risk of becoming violent, as are adolescents with antisocial, delinquent peers. These two types of peer relationships often go together, since adolescents who are rejected by, or unpopular with conventional peers, may find acceptance only in antisocial or delinquent peer groups. Social isolation—having neither conventional nor antisocial friends—is not a risk factor for violence, however. A third risk factor with a large effect size on violence is belonging to a gang. Gang membership increases the risk of violence above and beyond the risk posed by having delinquent peers. These three peer group factors appear to have independent effects, they sometimes cluster together, and they are all powerful late predictors of violence in adolescence.

Researchers who have studied what causes young people to join gangs have found that the risk factors for gang membership are virtually the same as those for violence generally. The notion that gangs act as surrogate families for children who do not have close ties to their own families is not borne out by recent data, but gangs do strengthen young people's sense of belonging, their independence from parents, and their self-esteem. Estimates from law enforcement agencies indicate that gang members are overwhelmingly male, and the great majority (almost 80 percent) is African American or Hispanic. However, surveys in which young people identify themselves as gang members suggest

♣ **It's A Fact!!**

Social disorganization is also a risk factor for violence in rural areas. One study of rural communities found that poverty plays a less important role in predicting violence than residential instability, broken homes, and other indicators of social disorganization. In fact, high residential instability, or a large proportion of broken homes, did not characterize very poor areas. In cities, however, the combination of poverty with instability and family disruption is predictive of violence.

Source: Office of the Surgeon General, U.S. Department of Health and Human Services, January 2001.

that there are substantially larger proportions of white and female gang members. In a survey of nearly 6,000 eighth graders in 1995, 25 percent of white students and 38 percent of female students reported they were gang members. Lacking comparisons within ethnic groups, it is difficult to tell whether ethnicity per se is a risk factor in gang membership.

Community: Increasing involvement in the community is a healthy part of adolescent development, unless the community itself poses a threat to health and safety. Social disorganization and the presence of crime and drugs in the neighborhood pose a small risk of violence when measured on an individual level. However, both of these risk factors have a substantially greater effect on the neighborhood level, where they measure the average rate of violent offending by youths living in the neighborhood or community.

Socially disorganized communities are characterized in part by economic and social flux, high turnover of residents, and a large proportion of disrupted or single-parent families, all of which lessen the likelihood that adults will be involved in informal networks of social control. As a result, there is generally little adult knowledge or supervision of the activities of teenagers and a high rate of crime. Moreover, in areas experiencing economic decline, there are likely to be few neighborhood businesses. In such an environment, it is hard for young people to avoid being drawn into violence. Not only are they on their own after school, they are exposed to violent adults and youth gangs, they have few part-time job opportunities, and their neighborhood is not likely to offer many after-school activities such as sports or youth groups.

Adolescents who are exposed to violence in their neighborhood feel vulnerable and unable to control their lives. These feelings can lead to helplessness and hopelessness. Such young people may turn to violence as a way of asserting control over their surroundings. They may arm themselves, or even join a gang, for protection. Studies have shown that adolescents exposed to violence are more likely to engage in violent acts, often as preemptive strikes in the face of a perceived threat.

Neighborhood adults who are involved in crime pose a risk because young people may emulate them. Easily available drugs add to the risk of violence. As noted earlier, drug use is associated with both a higher rate of offending and a longer criminal career. More important, ready availability of drugs indicates that considerable drug trafficking is taking place in the neighborhood, and drug trafficking is dangerous for buyer and seller alike.

Chapter 15

Warning Signs Of Youth Violence

Violence

It's the act of purposefully hurting someone. And it's a major issue facing today's young adults.

One in 12 high schoolers is threatened or injured with a weapon each year. If you're between the ages of 12 and 24, you face the highest risk of being the victim of violence.

At the same time, statistics show that by the early 1990s, the incidence of violence caused by young people reached unparalleled levels in American society.

There is no single explanation for the overall rise in youth violence. Many different factors cause violent behavior. The more these factors are present in your life, the more likely you are to commit an act of violence. Factors that contribute to violent behavior include:

• peer pressure

• need for attention or respect

• feelings of low self-worth

- early childhood abuse or neglect
- witnessing violence at home, in the community, or in the media
- easy access to weapons

Reasons For Violence

What causes someone to punch, kick, stab, or fire a gun at someone else or even him/herself?

There is never a simple answer to that question. But people often commit violence because of one or more of the following:

- **Expression:** Some people use violence to release feelings of anger or frustration. They think there are no answers to their problems and turn to violence to express their out of control emotions.

- **Manipulation:** Violence is used as a way to control others or get something they want.

- **Retaliation:** Violence is used to retaliate against those who have hurt them or someone they care about.

Violence is a learned behavior. Like all learned behaviors, it can be changed. This isn't easy, though. Since there is no single cause of violence, there is no one simple solution. The best you can do is learn to recognize the warning signs of violence and to get help when you see them in your friends or yourself.

Recognizing Violence Warning Signs In Others

Often people who act violently have trouble controlling their feelings. They may have been hurt by others. Some think that making people fear them through violence or threats of violence will solve their problems or earn them respect. This isn't true. People who behave violently lose respect. They find themselves isolated or disliked, and they still feel angry and frustrated.

If you see these immediate warning signs, violence is a serious possibility:

- loss of temper on a daily basis
- frequent physical fighting
- significant vandalism or property damage

- increase in use of drugs or alcohol

- increase in risk-taking behavior

- detailed plans to commit acts of violence

- announcing threats or plans for hurting others

- enjoying hurting animals

- carrying a weapon

If you notice the following signs over a period of time, the potential for violence exists:

- a history of violent or aggressive behavior

- serious drug or alcohol use

- gang membership or strong desire to be in a gang

- access to or fascination with weapons, especially guns

- threatening others regularly

- trouble controlling feelings like anger

- withdrawal from friends and usual activities

- feeling rejected or alone

- having been a victim of bullying

- poor school performance

- history of discipline problems or frequent run-ins with authority

- feeling constantly disrespected

- failing to acknowledge the feelings or rights of others

What You Can Do If Someone You Know Shows Violence Warning Signs

When you recognize violence warning signs in someone else, there are things you can do. Hoping that someone else will deal with the situation is the easy way out.

Above all, be safe. Don't spend time alone with people who show warning signs.

If possible, without putting yourself in danger, remove the person from the situation that's setting them off.

Tell someone you trust and respect about your concerns and ask for help. This could be a family member, guidance counselor, teacher, school psychologist, coach, clergy, school resource officer, or friend.

If you are worried about being a victim of violence, get someone in authority to protect you. Do not resort to violence or use a weapon to protect yourself.

The key to really preventing violent behavior is asking an experienced professional for help. The most important thing to remember is—don't go it alone.

Dealing With Anger

It's normal to feel angry or frustrated when you've been let down or betrayed.

But anger and frustration don't justify violent action. Anger is a strong emotion that can be difficult to keep in check, but the right response is always stay cool.

Here are some ways to deal with anger without resorting to violence:

- **Learn to talk about your feelings.** If you're afraid to talk, or if you can't find the right words to describe what you're going through, find a trusted friend or adult to help you one-on-one.

- **Express yourself calmly.** Express criticism, disappointment, anger, or displeasure without losing your temper or fighting. Ask yourself if your response is safe and reasonable.

- **Listen to others.** Listen carefully and respond without getting upset when someone gives you negative feedback. Ask yourself if you can really see the other person's point of view.

- **Negotiate.** Work out your problems with someone else by looking at alternative solutions and compromises.

Anger is part of life, but you can free yourself from the cycle of violence by learning to talk about your feelings. Be strong. Be safe. Be cool.

Are You At Risk For Violent Behavior?

If you recognize any of the warning signs for violent behavior in yourself, get help. You don't have to live with the guilt, sadness, and frustration that come from hurting others.

Admitting you have a concern about hurting others is the first step. The second is to talk to a trusted adult such as a school counselor or psychologist, teacher, family member, friend, or clergy. They can get you in touch with a licensed mental health professional who cares and can help.

Controlling Your Own Risk For Violent Behavior

Everyone feels anger in his or her own way. Start managing it by recognizing how anger feels to you.

✔ Quick Tip
How To Avoid Potentially Violent Situations

- Ignore insults or name-calling. It will be hard, but stay calm and do not let them see you sweat. Take a deep breath and try not to show that you are upset or angry. Above all, do not believe for one second what they are saying. Bullies feed on attention and are just trying to get a reaction from you. It is easier to give them the brush off if you do not let them get under your skin. They will get bored and move on.

- Avoid getting sucked into a scuffle, even if it means losing your stuff— your safety is way more important than your shoes. The only time you should ever fight back is when you have to defend yourself. Even then, keep your eyes open for an escape route. Chances are, if someone wants to fight, they know they have a good chance of winning.

- Do not be afraid to tell an adult if you are being bullied. You are not a snitch if you tell an adult you know that someone is hurting you. If you have tried to stop someone from bothering you and it is not working, get someone you trust involved to help you. If you see someone else in the same boat, find an adult to help. Get the problem out in the open. Once people know about it, the bully is no longer in control. Not telling anyone, especially because the bully told you not to, is just making him or her feel more powerful.

Source: Excerpted from "The Bully Roundup," Centers for Disease Control and Prevention (BAM! Body and Mind), 2003.

When you are angry, you probably feel:

- muscle tension
- accelerated heartbeat
- a "knot" or "butterflies" in your stomach
- changes in your breathing
- trembling
- goose bumps
- flushed in the face

You can reduce the rush of adrenaline that's responsible for your heart beating faster, your voice sounding louder, and your fists clenching if you:

- Take a few slow, deep breaths and concentrate on your breathing.
- Imagine yourself at the beach, by a lake, or anywhere that makes you feel calm and peaceful.
- Try other thoughts or actions that have helped you relax in the past.

Keep telling yourself:

- "Calm down."
- "I don't need to prove myself."
- "I'm not going to let him/her get to me."

Stop. Consider the consequences. Think before you act.

Try to find positive or neutral explanations for what that person did that provoked you.

Don't argue in front of other people.

Make your goal to defeat the problem, not the other person.

Learn to recognize what sets you off and how anger feels to you.

Learn to think through the benefits of controlling your anger and the consequences of losing control.

Most of all, stay cool and think. Only you have the power to control your own violent behavior. Don't let anger control you.

Chapter 16

Oppositional Defiant Disorder And Conduct Disorder

Oppositional Defiant Disorder

What is it?

Oppositional defiant disorder (ODD) is a psychiatric disorder that is characterized by two different sets of problems. These are aggressiveness and a tendency to purposefully bother and irritate others. It is often the reason that people seek treatment. When ODD is present with attention deficit hyperactivity disorder (ADHD), depression, Tourette syndrome, anxiety disorders, or other neuropsychiatric disorders, it makes life with that child far more difficult. For example, ADHD plus ODD is much worse than ADHD alone, often enough to make people seek treatment. The criteria for ODD are as follows:

• A pattern of negativistic, hostile, and defiant behavior lasting at least six months during which four or more of the following are present:

About This Chapter: Information under the heading "Oppositional Defiant Disorder" is excerpted from "Oppositional Defiant Disorder (ODD) and Conduct Disorder (CD) in Children and Adolescents: Diagnosis and Treatment," by James Chandler, MD, FRCPC. © 2006 James Chandler. Reprinted with permission. Text under the heading "Conduct Disorder," is excerpted from "Children and Adolescents with Conduct Disorder," National Mental Health Information Center, Substance Abuse and Mental Health Services Administration, U.S. Department of Health and Human Services, April 2003.

- often loses temper

- often argues with adults

- often actively defies or refuses to comply with adults' requests or rules

- often deliberately annoys people

- often blames others for his or her mistakes or misbehavior

- is often touchy or easily annoyed by others

- is often angry and resentful

- is often spiteful and vindictive

- The disturbance in behavior causes clinically significant impairment in social, academic, or occupational functioning.

How often is "often"?

All of the criteria above include the word "often". But what exactly does that mean? Recent studies have shown that these behaviors occur to a varying degree in all children. These researchers have found that the "often" is best solved by the following criteria:

- The following has occurred at all during the last three months:

  - is spiteful and vindictive

  - blames others for his or her mistakes or misbehavior

- The following occurs at least twice a week:

  - is touchy or easily annoyed by others

  - loses temper

  - argues with adults

  - actively defies or refuses to comply with adults' requests or rules

- The following occurs at least four times per week:

  - is angry and resentful

  - deliberately annoys people

What causes it?

Like most psychiatric illnesses, there are three main causes: environment, genetics, and medical problems. If the mother is smoking during her pregnancy, the child is two to three times more likely to end up with ODD when he is older.

The usual pattern is for problems to begin between ages one and three. If you think about it, a lot of these behaviors are normal at age two; but in this disorder, they never go away. It does run in families. If a parent is alcoholic and has been in trouble with the law, their children are almost three times as likely to have ODD. That is, 18% of children will have ODD if the parents are alcoholic and the father has been in trouble with the law.

How can you tell if a child has it?

ODD is diagnosed in the same way as many other psychiatric disorders in children. You need to examine the child, talk with the child, talk to the parents, and review the medical history. Sometimes other medical tests are necessary to make sure it is not something else. You always need to check children out for other psychiatric disorders, as it is common the children with ODD will have other problems, too.

Who gets it?

A lot of children. This is the most common psychiatric problem in children. Over 5% of children have this. In younger children it is more common in boys than girls, but as they grow older, the rate is the same in males and females.

What happens to children who have this when they grow up?

There are three main paths that a child will take.

First, there will be some lucky children who outgrow this. About half of children who have ODD as preschoolers will have no psychiatric problems at all by age eight.

Second, ODD may turn into something else. About 5–10% of preschoolers with ODD will eventually end up with ADHD and no signs of ODD at all. Other times ODD turns into conduct disorder (CD). This usually happens fairly early. That is, after three to four years of ODD, if it has not turned into CD, it won't ever. What predicts a child with ODD getting CD? A history of a biologic parent who was a career criminal and very severe ODD.

Third, the child may continue to have ODD without anything else. However, by the time preschoolers with ODD are eight years old, only 5% have ODD and nothing else.

Fourth, they continue to have ODD but add on comorbid anxiety disorders, comorbid ADHD, or comorbid depressive disorders. By the time these children are in the end of elementary school, about 25% will have mood or anxiety problems, which are disabling. That means that it is very important to watch for signs of mood disorder and anxiety, as children with ODD grow older.

Will children with ODD end up as criminals?

Probably not, unless they develop conduct disorder. Even then, many will grow out of it. Life may not be easy. People with ODD who are grown up often do best if they can work for themselves and stay away from alcohol. However, their tendency to irritate others often leads to a lonely life.

♣ It's A Fact!!
Oppositional Defiant Disorder
Rarely Travels Alone

It is exceptionally rare for a physician to see a child with only oppositional defiant disorder (ODD). Usually the child has some other neuropsychiatric disorder along with ODD. The tendency for disorders in medicine to occur together is called comorbidity. Understanding comorbidity in pediatric psychiatry is one of the most important areas of research at this moment.

If a child comes to a clinic and is diagnosed with attention deficit hyperactivity disorder, about 30–40% of the time the child will also have ODD.

Source: © 2006 James Chandler. Reprinted with permission.

What is the difference between ODD and ADHD?

ODD is characterized by aggressiveness, but not impulsiveness. In ODD people annoy you purposefully, while it is usually not so purposeful in ADHD. ODD signs and symptoms are much more difficult to live with than ADHD. Children with ODD can sit still.

What difference does it make if you have ADHD or ADHD plus ODD?

A lot. Children and adolescents with ADHD alone do things without thinking, but not necessarily oppositional things. An ADHD child may impulsively push someone too hard on a swing and knock the child down on the ground. She would likely be sorry she did this afterward. A child with ODD plus ADHD might push the kid out of the swing and say she did not do it.

Conduct Disorder

What is conduct disorder?

Children with conduct disorder repeatedly violate the personal or property rights of others and the basic expectations of society. A diagnosis of conduct disorder is likely when symptoms continue for six months or longer.

What are the signs of conduct disorder?

Symptoms of conduct disorder include the following:

* aggressive behavior that harms or threatens other people or animals

* destructive behavior that damages or destroys property

* lying or theft

* truancy or other serious violations of rules

* early tobacco, alcohol, and substance use and abuse

* precocious sexual activity

Children with conduct disorder or oppositional defiant disorder also may experience the following:

- higher rates of depression, suicidal thoughts, suicide attempts, and suicide

- academic difficulties

- poor relationships with peers or adults

- sexually transmitted diseases

- difficulty staying in adoptive, foster, or group homes

- higher rates of injuries, school expulsions, and problems with the law

✤ **It's A Fact!!**
Conduct disorder is known as a "disruptive behavior disorder" because of its impact on children and their families, neighbors, and schools.

Source: Substance Abuse and Mental Health Services Administration, 2003.

How common is conduct disorder?

Conduct disorder affects 1 to 4% of 9- to 17-year-olds, depending on exactly how the disorder is defined. The disorder appears to be more common in boys than in girls and more common in cities than in rural areas.

Who is at risk for conduct disorder?

Research shows that some cases of conduct disorder begin in early childhood, often by the preschool years. In fact, some infants who are especially "fussy"

☞ Remember!!

Although conduct disorder is one of the most difficult behavior disorders to treat, young people often benefit from a range of services that include the following:

- training for parents on how to handle child or adolescent behavior

- family therapy

- training in problem-solving skills for children or adolescents

- community-based services that focus on the young person within the context of family and community influences

Source: Substance Abuse and Mental Health Services Administration, 2003.

appear to be at risk for developing conduct disorder. Other factors that may make a child more likely to develop conduct disorder include the following:

- early maternal rejection
- separation from parents, without an adequate alternative caregiver
- early institutionalization
- family neglect
- abuse or violence
- parental mental illness
- parental marital discord
- large family size
- crowding
- poverty

Chapter 17

Media And Video Game Violence: Is There A Link To Violent Behavior?

The Violent Side Of Video Games

Scientists are discovering that playing video and computer games and watching TV and movies can change the way we act, think, and feel. Whether these changes are good or bad has become a subject of intense debate.

Concerns About Violence

Violence is one of the biggest concerns, especially as computer graphics and special effects become more realistic. Some parents and teachers blame school shootings and other aggressive behavior on media violence—as seen in TV programs, movies, and video games.

"If you've ever watched young children watching kickboxing," says child psychologist John Murray, "within a few minutes they start popping up and pushing and shoving and imitating the actions." Murray is at Kansas State University in Manhattan, Kansas.

About This Chapter: This chapter begins with text from "The Violent Side Of Video Games," reprinted with permission from *Science News for Kids*, © 2004; and continues with text from "What Video Games Can Teach Us," reprinted with permission from *Science News for Kids*, © 2004.

There's also evidence that people become less sensitive to violence after a while, Murray says. In other words, you get so used to seeing it that you eventually think it's not such a big deal.

Then there's the "mean world syndrome." If you watch lots of violence, you may start to think the world is a bad place. You may sometimes have trouble falling asleep if you watch the news on TV or read the newspaper right before going to bed.

Still, it's hard to prove that violence on TV leads to violence in real life. It might be possible, for example, that people who are already aggressive for other reasons are more drawn to violent games and TV shows.

Brain Clues

To try to make the link between seeing violence and acting violently, Murray is looking for clues in the brain.

In his most recent study, eight boys and girls between the ages of 8 and 12 watched a series of video clips. Some clips showed violent fighting scenes of Sylvester Stallone from the movie *Rocky IV*. Other clips were full of action, but no violence. Others were just blank screens. During the experiment, each kid lay inside a special brain-imaging machine. Such a machine takes pictures of the brain and shows which parts of the brain are working at different times.

✎ What's It Mean?

Amygdala: A discrete brain area that is part of the limbic system, has a large number of dopamine-containing neurons, and plays a role in the learning and performing of certain behaviors in response to incentive stimuli (i.e., motivation, reinforcement).

Source: "Treatment for Stimulant Use Disorders, *Treatment Improvement Protocol (TIP) Series 33*, Appendix D Glossary, Center for Substance Abuse Treatment, Substance Abuse and Mental Health Services Administration, U.S. Department of Health and Human Services, 1999.

Murray and his colleagues found that exposure to violent video clips activated the amygdala, a thumbnail-sized area in the brain. The right side was particularly active.

The amygdala is best known as the "fight or flight" organ. It senses danger and prepares you to either go to battle or run away. Your breathing slows down. You become hyper-aware of movements in the environment. And blood rushes to your brain's core, among other effects.

"If someone drops a snake in front of you, most people . . . gasp," Murray says. "That's actually the amygdala responding."

Video Power

Most of the research has focused on TV and movie violence, mainly because TV and movies have been around much longer than video games, says psychologist Craig Anderson of Iowa State University in Ames, Iowa. Anderson has a Web site dedicated to looking at the link between video games and violence.

In his own research and in analyses of research by others, Anderson says that he has detected a connection between violent video games and violent behavior. He has found that people who repeatedly play violent games have aggressive thoughts and become less helpful and sociable. Physically, their heart rates accelerate.

Video games might have an even more powerful effect on the brain than TV does, Murray says. Players actively participate in the violence. In games like *Grand Theft Auto 3*, for example, the goal is to kill as many people as you can. The more violent you are, the more points you win.

Next time you play a violent video game, Murray suggests, check your pulse just before and after each round as one way to see how the game affects you.

"Ninety-nine percent of the time, I'll bet your heart rate will have increased rather dramatically while playing one," Murray says. "This indicates that . . . you are being affected."

Three teenagers from Puerto Rico have data to back up that observation. At the International Science and Engineering Fair in Cleveland in 2003,

Wildaliz Arias Perez, Derek Mercado Rivera, and Jacqueline Velez Gonzales presented a study looking at how video games affect people.

With the help of a school nurse, the high school seniors found that people of all ages showed a rise in blood pressure and heart rate after playing the super violent game *Capcom vs. SNK Pro*. Playing *Super Bust-A-Move 2*, an active, nonviolent game, did not have the same effect.

Kids in Puerto Rico are addicted to video games just like in the United States, Derek said, and he worries about the consequences. "So many kids have to play all day, like more than 4 hours," he said.

Not so fast, some researchers say. Although violent video games increase a person's heart rate and blood pressure, it doesn't necessarily follow that such games make a person more violent. It might not be fair to blame all—or even a part—of society's problems on media violence, these critics say.

✤ It's A Fact!!

There's more to video games than just violent content. In fact, a variety of studies are starting to show that playing video games can actually help people develop visual skills, learn about computers, and stay interested in school.

Source: "The Violent Side Of Video Games," reprinted with permission from *Science News for Kids*, © 2004.

What Video Games Can Teach Us

Here's some news for you to share with your parents and teachers: Video games might actually be good for you.

Whenever a wave of teenage violence strikes, movies, TV, or video games often take the heat. Some adults assume that movies, TV, and video games are a bad influence on kids, and they blame these media for causing various problems. A variety of studies appear to support the link between media violence and bad behavior among kids.

But media don't necessarily cause violence, says James Gee. Gee is an education professor at the University of Wisconsin, Madison. "You get a group of teenage boys who shoot up a school—of course they've played video games," Gee says. "Everyone does. It's like blaming food because we have obese people."

Video games are innocent of most of the charges against them, Gee says. The games might actually do a lot of good. Gee has written a book titled *What Video Games Have to Teach Us About Learning and Literacy.*

A growing number of researchers agree with Gee. If used in the right way, video and computer games have the potential to inspire learning. And they can help players improve coordination and visual skills.

Attention-Getting Games

A good video game is challenging, entertaining, and complicated, Gee says. It usually takes 50 to 60 hours of intense concentration to finish one. Even kids who can't sit still in school can spend hours trying to solve a video or computer game.

"Kids diagnosed with ADHD because they can't pay attention will play games for 9 straight hours on the computer," Gee says. "The game focuses attention in a way that school doesn't."

The captivating power of video games might lie in their interactive nature. Players don't just sit and watch. They get to participate in the action and solve problems. Some games even allow players to make changes in the game, allowing new possibilities.

And kids who play computer games often end up knowing more about computers than their parents do. "Kids today are natives in a culture in which their parents are immigrants," Gee says.

In his 2 to 3 years of studying the social influences of video games, Gee has seen a number of young gamers become computer science majors in college. One kid even ended up as a teaching assistant during his freshman year because the school's computer courses were too easy for him.

Screen Reading

Video games can enhance reading skills, too. In the game *Animal Crossing*, for instance, players become characters who live in a town full of animals. Over the course of the game, you can buy a house, travel from town to town, go to museums, and do other ordinary things. All the while, you're writing notes to other players and talking to the animals. Because kids are interested in the game, they often end up reading at a level well above their grade, even if they say they don't like to read.

Games can inspire new interests. After playing a game called *Age of Mythology*, Gee says, kids (like his 8-year-old son) often start checking out mythology books from the library or join internet chat groups about mythological characters. History can come alive to a player participating in the game.

Even violent games have a positive side, Gee says. "*Grand Theft Auto 3* does not exist to get off on shooting people," he says. When the game begins, your character has just been released from jail. You need to figure out how to make a living, but the only people you know are criminals. Along the way, you might end up fighting or killing people, but you don't have to.

"The game offers you a palette of choices," Gee says. Players must confront moral dilemmas, develop social relationships, and solve challenging problems that might apply to real life, he says. "How compelling would a game be if you only had good choices?"

Improved Skills

Video games might also help improve visual skills. That was what researchers from the University of Rochester in New York recently found.

In the study, frequent game players between the ages of 18 and 23 were better at monitoring what was happening around them than those who didn't play as often or didn't play at all. They could keep track of more objects at a time. And they were faster at picking out objects from a cluttered environment.

"Above and beyond the fact that action video games can be beneficial," says Rochester neuroscientist Daphne Bavelier, "our findings are surprising because they show that the learning induced by video game playing occurs quite fast and generalizes outside the gaming experience."

The research might lead to better ways to train soldiers or treat people with attention problems, the researchers say, though they caution against taking that point too far.

♣ It's A Fact!!

Researchers at the Massachusetts Institute of Technology have started a project they describe as the "Education Arcade." The project brings together researchers, scholars, game designers and others interested in developing and using computer games in the classroom.

Source: "What Video Games Can Teach Us," reprinted with permission from *Science News for Kids*, © 2004.

Says Bavelier, "We certainly don't mean to convey the message that kids can play video games instead of doing their homework!"

If Gee gets his way, though, teachers might some day start incorporating computer games into their assignments. Already, scientists and the military use computer games to help simulate certain situations for research or training, he says. Why shouldn't schools do the same thing?

"Kids are beginning to see school as really out of step with culture," Gee says. Making computer technology part of the learning experience could change all that.

Some kids already go to educational Web sites where they can interact with other kids and help solve problems. At *Whyville* (www.whyville.net), for example, kids from all over the world can chat, build an online identity, and learn math and science as they roam a virtual world.

Looking at the bright side of video and computer games could also help bring kids and adults closer together. Playing games can be a social activity, during which kids and adults learn from each other. By opening up lines of communication and understanding, maybe one day we'll praise video games for saving society, not blame them for destroying it.

On the one hand, there's still a lot more to learn about how video games really affect us. On the other hand, there's also a lot to learn about how to harness them for our benefit.

Chapter 18

Animal Abuse And Youth Violence

What is animal cruelty?

Animal cruelty encompasses a range of behaviors harmful to animals, from neglect to malicious killing. Most cruelty investigated by humane officers is unintentional neglect that can be resolved through education. Intentional cruelty, or abuse, is knowingly depriving an animal of food, water, shelter, socialization, or veterinary care, or maliciously torturing, maiming, mutilating, or killing an animal.

Why is it a concern?

All animal cruelty is a concern because it is wrong to inflict suffering on any living creature. Intentional cruelty is a particular concern because it is a sign of psychological distress and often indicates that an individual either has already experienced violence or may be predisposed to committing acts of violence.

Is there any evidence of a connection between animal cruelty and human violence?

Absolutely. Many studies in psychology, sociology, and criminology during the last 25 years have demonstrated that violent offenders frequently

About This Chapter: Information in this chapter is excerpted from "Frequently Asked Questions about Animal Cruelty" and "Children and Animal Cruelty: What Parents Should Know." Text in this chapter is reprinted with permission from The Humane Society of the United States, www.humanesociety.org. © 2007 The Humane Society of the United States. All rights reserved.

have childhood and adolescent histories of serious and repeated animal cruelty. The Federal Bureau of Investigation (FBI) has recognized the connection since the 1970s when its analysis of the lives of serial killers suggested that most had killed or tortured animals as children. Other research has shown consistent patterns of animal cruelty among perpetrators of more common forms of violence including child abuse, spouse abuse, and elder abuse. In fact, the American Psychiatric Association considers animal cruelty one of the diagnostic criteria of conduct disorder.

♣ It's A Fact!!
Violent Marriages May Make Violent Children

Children of violent marriages may be more than twice as likely to set fires intentionally or be cruel to animals than those from nonviolent homes, according to new research.

The study shows that problems in the family, especially violent behavior among father figures, significantly increase the risk of fire setting and animal cruelty in children, and these behaviors set the stage for later adolescent delinquency.

Researchers say childhood fire setting and animal cruelty may be linked to childhood psychological problems such as attention deficit hyperactivity disorder (ADHD) or conduct disorder, which may lead to later chronic criminal behavior, but few studies have looked at the relationship between these behaviors and family risk factors.

This study suggests that the relationship between fire setting and animal cruelty and juvenile delinquency is potentially strong, and any sign of these behaviors should be taken seriously and addressed at an early age.

Family Factors Tied To Fire Setting And Animal Cruelty

In the study, researchers followed a group of about 300 battered women and their children for ten years and asked them periodically about family life and any problem behavior in their children.

The results appear in the July 2004 issue of the *Journal of the American Academy of Child and Adolescent Psychiatry*.

The study showed that children from homes with violent marriages were 2.4 times more likely to set fires than those residing in nonviolent homes. Children

Why would anyone be cruel to animals?

There can be many reasons. Animal cruelty, like any other form of violence, is often committed by a person who feels powerless, unnoticed, and under the control of others. The motive may be to shock, threaten, intimidate, or offend others, or to demonstrate rejection of society's rules. Some who are cruel to animals copy things they have seen or that have been done to them. Others see harming an animal as a safe way to get revenge on someone who cares about that animal.

from homes where the mother's partner harmed pets or drank large quantities of alcohol were also more likely to engage in fire-setting behavior.

In addition, researchers found that children from violent homes were 2.3 times more likely to be cruel to animals, and harsh parenting from either parent also increased the risk of animal cruelty.

Over time, the study showed that children who set fires were nearly four times more likely than non-fire setters to be referred to juvenile court in adolescence, and they were nearly five times as likely be arrested for a violent crime.

The researchers did not find a relationship between childhood cruelty to animals and a referral to juvenile court for an offense. However, animal abusers were twice as likely to commit a violent offense such as assault or possession of a weapon.

The researchers show that a diagnosis of conduct disorder was more than six times higher in children who set fires and more than five times higher in children who abuse animals.

"These findings converge with those from other studies generally linking family dysfunction and childhood conduct disorders," write researcher Kimberly D. Becker, PhD, of the University of Hawaii, and colleagues. "An intriguing finding is that most of the significant family variables were associated with partner behavior."

"Future research should investigate the mechanisms by which a violent antisocial man in the home contributes to a child's fire setting and animal cruelty," they write.

Source: "Violent Marriages May Make Violent Children," Copyright 2004 by WebMD. Reproduced with permission of WebMD via the Copyright Clearance Center.

As natural "explorers," don't all children sometimes harm animals?

Absolutely not. While some children kill insects, few torture pets or other small creatures. If allowed to harm animals, children are more likely to be violent later in life. Animal cruelty, like any other violence, should never be attributed to a stage of development.

What kind of children are cruel to animals?

Serious or repeated animal cruelty is seen more often in boys than in girls. Children as young as four may harm animals, but such behavior is most common during adolescence. Cruelty is often associated with children who do poorly in school and have low self-esteem and few friends. Children who are cruel to animals are often characterized as bullies and may have a history of truancy, vandalism, and other antisocial behaviors.

What does animal cruelty indicate about family dynamics?

Researchers say that a child's violence against animals often represents displaced hostility and aggression stemming from neglect or abuse of the child or of another family member. Animal cruelty committed by any member of a family, whether parent or child, often means child abuse occurs in that family.

♣ It's A Fact!!

In a review of 1,677 animal cruelty cases from 2001, The Humane Society of the United States found that teens were responsible for 20 percent of those involving deliberate abuse. And of that group, 95 percent were young men. The most common offenses included burning and shooting animals. These findings raise concern not only for the animals who suffer at the hands of teens, but also for the young people who commit these terrible acts. Without proper intervention, they may be at risk for escalating their violence toward people.

Source: Excerpted from "Teaching Teens Compassion: First Strike® reaches out to teens." Text is reprinted with permission from The Humane Society of the United States, www.humanesociety.org. © 2007 The Humane Society of the United States. All rights reserved.

Chapter 19

Teen Drug Use And Violence

Drug Use And Violence

Teenagers abuse a variety of drugs, both legal and illegal. Some of the most commonly used drugs include alcohol, marijuana, inhalants, stimulants (cocaine, crack, and speed), LSD, PCP, prescription medications, opiates, heroin, steroids, tobacco, and club drugs, like ecstasy (MDMA).

For teenagers, is there a strong relationship between the use of drugs and violence?

Teens who report engaging in violent behavior are also extremely likely to report using drugs. One national survey found that 85 percent of violent teens reported using marijuana, and 55 percent reported using several illegal drugs.

Do drugs cause teens to be violent?

The relationship between drugs and violence is complicated.

About This Chapter: Information under the heading "Drug Use And Violence" is from "Teen Drug Use And Violence," National Youth Violence Prevention Resource Center, 2002. Text under the heading "Drug-Facilitated Sexual Assault," is excerpted from "Drug-Facilitated Sexual Assault Fast Facts: Questions and Answers," National Drug Intelligence Center, a component of the U.S. Department of Justice, April 2004.

Some teens may become violent under the influence of drugs. It is also likely that some teens engage in violence to get money to buy drugs. In most cases, however, it appears that the use of drugs does not cause violent behavior.

Instead, it seems that violence and the use of drugs are both part of a lifestyle that involves antisocial and delinquent behavior. In many cases, the violent behavior actually comes before the drug use. The drug use is just one aspect of a risky and dangerous lifestyle.

Do teens who use drugs also tend to engage in other behaviors that put them at risk?

Almost 90 percent of the teens who use drugs also do other things that put them or those around them at risk for serious harm including drinking heavily, fighting, carrying weapons, and having unsafe sex.

Children under the age of 12 that experiment with drugs are at a much greater risk than other children for engaging in serious violence during their teenage years, probably because the use of illegal drugs is an early sign of antisocial attitudes and involvement in delinquent behavior.

While the use of drugs does not generally cause teens to become involved in violence, those violent teens who do use illegal drugs tend to engage in violent behavior more frequently and to continue to engage in violence much longer than those violent teens who do not use drugs.

♣ It's A Fact!!
Get The Facts About Drugs

Many teens are not aware of basic facts about drugs and how drugs can affect their brains and bodies. For example, did you know the following facts:

- Ecstasy, or MDMA, can affect users' brains, causing problems that interfere with normal learning and memory.

- Even first-time crack or cocaine users can have seizures or heart attacks, which can kill them.

- Marijuana damages the lungs and makes the body less able to resist illnesses.

Sometimes, watching television or listening to people talk, it is easy to believe that everyone is smoking marijuana or trying other drugs. In fact, most teens have not tried marijuana or other drugs, and using them does not make you "cool." If someone offers you drugs, just say, "No thanks," or "I'm not into that." You may want to try suggesting another activity instead.

Source: National Youth Violence Prevention Resource Center, 2002.

Are teens who use drugs more likely to attempt and die by suicide?

Research has not proven that drug use actually causes suicidal behavior, only that the two behaviors are associated. It may be that teens who have emotional problems are more likely to use drugs and to contemplate suicide. Another possibility is that the use of drugs aggravates pre-existing depression or other emotional problems. Drugs may also impair the judgment of teens considering suicide, making suicide attempts more likely.

How can a teen recognize signs of a drug problem in someone?

If a friend has one or more of the following warning signs, he or she may have a problem with drugs:

- getting high on a regular basis
- lying about the amount of drugs he or she is using
- believing that drugs are necessary to have fun
- constantly talking about using drugs
- feeling run-down, depressed, or even suicidal
- having problems at school or getting in trouble with the law
- giving up activities he or she used to do, such as playing sports or doing homework, and shunning friends who do not use drugs

If you recognize these signs in a friend or yourself, professional help may be necessary. Do not try to handle this on your own. Talk with an adult you can trust such as your parents or a trusted family member, a teacher, a school counselor, your clergy, or a professional at a mental health center.

Drug-Facilitated Sexual Assault

What is drug-facilitated sexual assault?

Drug-facilitated sexual assault involves the administration of an anesthesia-type drug to render a victim physically incapacitated or helpless and thus incapable of giving or withholding consent. Victims may be unconscious during all or parts of the sexual assault, and upon regaining consciousness, may experience anterograde amnesia—the inability to recall events that occurred while under the influence of the drug.

♣ **It's A Fact!!**
Alcohol And Dating Violence

Because 11 million drinkers are underage, alcohol plays a large part in many teenage abusive situations. More than 60 percent of sexual assaults will involve alcohol. In fact, one in four teenagers will experience sexual or nonsexual abuse by the time they finish college. Teenagers and women in their twenties are at higher risk of sexual abuse and verbal abuse than older women.

Although there have been many studies on domestic violence experienced by adult women, studies on domestic violence experienced by younger women in high school and college are just beginning. Despite increased public awareness about drinking and abuse, many people still do not realize that violence and problem drinking occur in younger relationships.

Dating behavior in high school and college helps to define the relationships men and women will have as adults. If the man in earlier relationships is violent and uses alcohol, he has a greater chance of being violent again later in life. If a young woman encounters violence early in her dating experience, she is more likely to experience it again when she is older.

Source: Excerpted from "Alcohol and Dating Violence," from the online course titled "Silence Hurts: Alcohol Abuse and Violence Against Women," Substance Abuse and Mental Health Services Administration, U.S. Department of Health and Human Services, June 2004.

How prevalent are drug-facilitated sexual assaults?

There are no conclusive estimates as to the number of drug-facilitated sexual assaults that occur each year; however, nationwide law enforcement reporting indicates that the number of such assaults appears to be increasing. Many drug-facilitated sexual assaults are not reported. Victims often are reluctant to report incidents because of a sense of embarrassment, guilt, or perceived responsibility, or because they lack specific recall of the assault. Moreover, most of the drugs typically used in the commission of sexual assaults are rapidly absorbed and metabolized by the body, thereby rendering them undetectable in routine urine and blood drug screenings.

What drugs are used in the commission of drug-facilitated sexual assaults?

Sexual assaults have long been linked to the abuse of substances, primarily alcohol, that may decrease inhibitions and render the user incapacitated. In addition to alcohol, the drugs most often implicated in the commission of drug-facilitated sexual assaults are GHB, Rohypnol (a benzodiazepine), ketamine, and Soma, although others, including other benzodiazepines and other sedative hypnotics, are used as well. These drugs often render victims unconscious—an effect that is quickened and intensified when the drugs are taken with alcohol. A person also may become a victim after taking such a drug willingly. Because of the sedative properties of these drugs, victims often have no memory of an assault, only an awareness or sense that they were violated.

Where do perpetrators obtain drugs used to facilitate sexual assaults?

Drugs used in sexual assaults typically are distributed at raves, dance clubs, and bars, but they are increasingly being sold in schools, on college campuses, and at private parties. Some of these drugs also are purchased via the internet while others, particularly prescription benzodiazepines, are often found in homes. Law enforcement reporting indicates that these drugs are widely available in most urban areas and are becoming increasingly available in suburban and rural communities.

Is drug-facilitated sexual assault illegal?

Yes, drug-facilitated sexual assault is illegal. Most of the drugs typically used to facilitate sexual assaults—GHB, ketamine, and Rohypnol—are designated as controlled substances under the Controlled Substances Act of 1970. The Drug-Induced Rape Prevention and Punishment Act of 1996 (Public Law 104-305) modified 21 U.S.C. § 841 to provide penalties of up to 20 years imprisonment and fines for persons who intend to commit a crime of violence (including rape) by distributing a controlled substance to another individual without that individual's knowledge.

Chapter 20

The Relationship Between Substance Abuse And Violence Against Women

Facts About Substance Abuse And Violence Against Women

- Regular alcohol abuse is one of the leading risk factors for intimate partner violence.

- Attackers who abuse alcohol most frequently tend to commit more severe sexual assaults than those who do not abuse alcohol.

- The relationship between alcohol and drug abuse and abuse of women is strongest for those men who already believe that male power and control over a woman are acceptable in certain situations.

About This Chapter: Information in this chapter is from "Facts About Substance Abuse and Violence Against Women," "The Complicated Relationship Between Substance Abuse and Violence," "Motives for Alcohol and Drug Use and Violence," "Myths and Facts About Substance Abuse and Violence Against Women," "The Connection Between Drug and Alcohol Abuse and Violence Against Women," "Substance Abuse and the Violent Partner," and "Effects of Substance Abuse and Violence on Children," excerpted from *It Won't Happen to Me: Substance Abuse-Related Violence Against Women for Anyone Concerned about the Issues,* Prevention Pathways Online Course, Center for Substance Abuse Prevention, Substance Abuse and Mental Health Administration, U. S. Department of Health and Human Services, 2004.

- A national survey of female college students found that 15 percent were raped at some time since age 14. In 64 percent of these cases, the offender was drinking, and in 53 percent of the cases, the victim was drinking.

- Abused women of all races reported higher stress, less support from partners, less support from others, lower self-esteem, and increased substance abuse.

- Drinking by offenders and victims is associated with assaults occurring in social situations (such as bars, parties) in which the victim does not know the offender well before the assault.

- A woman drinking alcohol may increase her risk of sexual assault. Attackers may interpret a woman's drinking as sexual consent, and this can lead to later assault. Assailants may also believe that women who do not strongly resist their advances are, therefore, agreeing to have sex.

- Alcohol use precedes acts of domestic violence in 25 to 50 percent of all cases.

The Complicated Relationship Between Substance Abuse And Violence

The relationship between substance abuse and violence against women is complicated. Although some people believe that drugs and alcohol cause violence, they do not. However, alcohol or drug use can increase the risk of violence. It also affects how often violence occurs and how severe it is.

For example, a man with a short temper may be more likely to release his anger onto his partner when he is intoxicated. He may also do greater harm to the woman when he has been drinking. Alcohol can also impair impulse control.

Part of the problem in addressing substance-related violence against women stems from difficulty dealing with alcohol and drugs. Attempts to prohibit alcohol use have failed, and alcohol use has become common in American society. Unfortunately, alcohol use is often used to excuse harmful behavior. Many men try to blame their violence on their drinking.

Motives For Alcohol And Drug Use And Violence

Alcohol is the most widely used and abused drug in the United States. Fourteen million people in the United States have alcohol problems. Still, many people do not think that alcohol is a drug or that it is harmful. However, even in small doses, alcohol can affect our judgment and behavior. Often, it leads to violence.

Alcohol or drugs may be used to do the following:

• experience feelings of relaxation or happiness

• fight stress or to take away feelings of sadness or depression

• enhance performance

• "expand the mind" by changing the perception of reality

• numb feelings of guilt, shame, anger, or loneliness

Similarly, violence may make a person feel better by allowing him or her to do the following:

• release feelings of stress

• vent anger or frustration

• avoid painful issues

• shift blame

• feel more in control

> ### ♣ It's A Fact!!
> In some cases, individuals may be at risk for alcohol or drug abuse and violence due to a combination of risk factors. Difficulty coping with life or controlling negative feelings can contribute both to substance abuse and violence.

Myths And Facts About Substance Abuse And Violence Against Women

Myth: Substance abuse causes a man to become violent.

Fact: Many men use this excuse after a violent incident. Not all substance abusers are violent. Not all violent people abuse alcohol or drugs. When a man is under the influence of a substance, the chance of his acting out aggressive or violent tendencies is increased. With his inhibitions lowered, the man may act before thinking. While substance abuse and violence often occur together, one does not cause the other. Because substance abuse does not cause violence in the home or any other violence against women, requiring violent people to attend only substance abuse treatment programs will not effectively end the violence.

Myth: A girl would know if "date rape" drugs (Rohypnol, gamma-hydroxybutyrate (GHB), or ketamine) had been put in her drink.

Fact: Rohypnol, GHB, and ketamine are called "date rape" drugs because they are colorless, odorless, and tasteless. This means that if a man puts the drug in a woman's drink at a bar or party, she will not know it is in there unless she sees him put the drug in her drink. If a woman leaves to go to the restroom or talk to another friend, the man has plenty of time to slip the drug into her drink.

Myth: Very few women are abused in our country.

Fact: Abuse of a woman occurs about every 15 seconds in the United States. An estimated three to four million women in America are beaten each year by their husbands or partners.

Myth: Alcoholism and domestic abuse do not have anything in common.

Fact: They do share a few characteristics: (1) Both may be passed from generation to generation, (2) Both involve denying there is a problem and trying to make the problem less important than it is, and (3) Both involve isolation of the family.

Myth: Violence against women by an intimate partner is only a momentary loss of control. It rarely happens more than once.

Fact: According to the American Medical Association, 47 percent of men who beat their wives, girlfriends, or mothers do so at least three times per year.

Myth: Victims of repeated violence must have a mental illness or are crazy.

Fact: This mistaken idea goes back to the belief that anyone would be crazy or "sick" to take the abuse. Most female victims are not mentally ill, although those who are ill are certainly not protected from abuse from their partners or intimates. There are many reasons a woman does not just "leave" a violent situation. Some victims of violence suffer psychological effects, such as posttraumatic stress disorder, substance abuse, or depression.

Some reasons a woman may not leave a violent situation include the following:

- dependence on her partner's money or earnings
- fear, shame, guilt
- family pressure to keep the marriage "intact"
- cultural or religious reasons
- children
- not having any place to go
- being socially isolated (abuser keeps the woman from interacting with friends and family so that she is emotionally dependent only on him)

Myth: Once a woman is abused, she will never leave the abuser.

Fact: Most women do leave the violent conditions, although it may take several attempts to do so. Victims who seek and receive legal assistance at an early stage increase their chances of obtaining the protection they need to leave their abusers. A woman may have many reasons for waiting or for making several tries before leaving for good. The most dangerous time for a woman is immediately after she leaves the abusive home. Therefore, it is important for the woman to get help planning to leave safely.

Myth: Violence against women does not happen to older or disabled women.

Fact: Any woman can become a victim of violence. The following are some examples:

- A teenager or young woman (ages 12 to 24) may be sexually or physically assaulted or abused by a stranger, acquaintance, romantic partner, or family member.
- A woman (ages 25 to 55) may be assaulted or abused by her husband or ex-husband, boyfriend, partner, acquaintance, or stranger.
- A woman who works outside the home may be assaulted or abused by a coworker.
- An older woman (55 or older) may be assaulted or abused by her children, husband or ex-husband, caregiver, or a stranger.
- Older and disabled women are often dependent on their family for support, shelter, and daily living requirements (e.g., medicine). Abuse may be

physical or it may come in the form of "neglect" by the family member withholding assistance or food. This type of abuse goes largely unreported.

Myth: Women ask for rape by how they act or dress.

Fact: Women do not want to be raped. How a woman dresses or acts does not give a man permission to rape her. No means no.

Myth: All rapists are sexually perverted or psychotic.

Fact: Rape is a violent crime brought about by the need for power and control, not sex. Men who are misinformed about women or sex, or who can only express their feelings of weakness, pain, and rage through sexual assault, commit the most rapes.

Myth: Men and women are the victims of intimate partner violence in equal numbers.

Fact: Women make up nearly 85 percent of victims of all intimate partner violence. Twenty-two percent of all violent acts against women were from an intimate, whereas only three percent of violent acts against men were from an intimate.

Myth: Very little of the violence against women is actually from an intimate partner.

Fact: According to the National Institute of Justice and the Centers for Disease Control and Prevention, 76 percent of the women who were raped and/or physically assaulted since age 18 were assaulted by a current or former husband, a partner with whom they live, or a date, compared with 18 percent of the men.

The Connection Between Drug And Alcohol Abuse And Violence Against Women

The connection between drug and alcohol abuse and violence against women can take many forms and involve many factors. For example, some men may feel a need for power and control. This need may lead to alcohol or drug use to escape feelings of low self-esteem. It can also lead to violence to gain control.

The same need may be filled in different ways. In some cases, a man could abuse alcohol or drugs and become violent. Substance use could exacerbate violent tendencies. Some women may feel a loss of power and control related to violent victimization. They may turn to alcohol or drugs to escape feelings of helplessness, shame, guilt, and pain. Others may have a drinking problem, which can put them at greater risk of becoming victims of violence.

If the man drinks or uses drugs, he may force her to join him, threatening violence if she does not. In addition, some men may force women to use alcohol or drugs in order to lower their resistance. Thus, drug and alcohol abuse can play a role in violence before, during, or after an incident.

Substance Abuse And The Violent Partner

Not all men with alcohol or drug problems become violent, just as not all violent men abuse alcohol or drugs. However, alcohol and drug use remain major risk factors for violent behavior. The percentage of batterers who are under the influence of alcohol when they assault their partners ranges from 48 percent to 87 percent. Most research indicates a 60 to 70 percent rate of alcohol abuse and a 13 to 20 percent rate of drug abuse.

♣ **It's A Fact!!**
Impaired judgment from alcohol use may lead a woman to engage in risky behavior.

For men, being physically abused as a child is linked to substance abuse as an adult. In addition, men who witness or are victims of violence in the home as a child may copy the violence later. They may become abusive when angry or frustrated. These men may not have learned nonviolent ways of expressing their feelings.

Approximately 46 percent of men who commit acts of intimate partner violence also have substance abuse problems. They have to work on stopping their violence as well as their addiction. If they are treated only for the addiction, the violence will continue.

In fact, many victims report that during their partner's recovery or sobriety, the abuse continues. Often, it gets worse. This can create more danger than before the sobriety. In some cases, victims report that physical violence decreases. However, other forms of control such as threats, manipulation, and isolation increase.

Thus, men who are violent and abuse substances need treatment for both conditions at the same time. This approach can improve the victim's safety and help prevent the abuser from going back to drugs or alcohol. The more violent he becomes when sober, the more likely he will be to use drugs or alcohol again.

Effects Of Substance Abuse And Violence On Children

Alcohol and drug abuse, when coupled with violence, doubles the need for denial. This can create an even greater sense of hopelessness for family members. Unfortunately, children at very young ages witness the violence and substance abuse and end up suffering the effects.

In addition to witnessing violence, children may experience it. In one survey of more than 6,000 American families, 50 percent of men who frequently assaulted their wives also frequently abused their children.

♣ **It's A Fact!!**
At least 3.3 million children between the ages of 3 and 19 are at risk of being hurt by parental violence every year.

Children may not see the violence, but they often hear it and see the results. From a hiding place, children may hear their parents yelling, crying, and screaming. They may hear the sound of threats, physical blows, or glass breaking.

Children may see the results of abuse in torn clothing, bloody bruises on the mother's face or body, broken furniture, or wounded animals. The children run the risk of being injured either intentionally by the male hurting them or unintentionally by trying to protect their mother.

In any case, children living with violence can suffer lasting emotional trauma and react with shock, fear, and guilt. In addition, witnessing violence and living with violence can place children at risk for alcohol problems. More than five million youth in the United States under the age of 21 drink alcohol to excess, consuming five or more drinks in a row.

Chapter 21

Teen Dating Violence

What Is It?

Dating violence is controlling, abusive, and aggressive behavior in a romantic relationship. It can happen in straight or gay relationships. It can include verbal, emotional, physical, or sexual abuse, or a combination.

Controlling behavior may include the following.

- Not letting you hang out with your friends

- Calling or paging you frequently to find out where you are, whom you're with, and what you're doing

- Telling you what to wear

- Having to be with you all the time

Verbal and emotional abuse may include the following.

- Calling you names

- Jealousy

- Belittling you (cutting you down)

About This Chapter: Information in this chapter is from "Dating Violence," Teen Tools Fact Sheet, © 2007 National Center for Victims of Crime. All rights reserved. Reprinted with permission. To view the complete text of this fact sheet, including references, or for additional information about teen dating violence, visit www.ncvc.org.

• Threatening to hurt you, someone in your family, or himself or herself if you don't do what he or she wants

Physical abuse may include the following.

• Shoving   • Punching

• Slapping   • Pinching

• Hitting   • Kicking

• Hair pulling   • Strangling

Sexual abuse may include the following.

• Unwanted touching and kissing

• Forcing you to have sex

• Not letting you use birth control

• Forcing you to do other sexual things

If You Are A Victim Of Dating Violence, You Might...

• Think it's your fault.

• Feel angry, sad, lonely, depressed, or confused.

• Feel helpless to stop the abuse.

• Feel threatened or humiliated.

• Feel anxious.

• Not know what might happen next.

• Feel like you can't talk to family and friends.

• Be afraid of getting hurt more seriously.

• Feel protective of your boyfriend or girlfriend.

You're Not Alone

• One in five teens in a serious relationship report having been hit, slapped, or pushed by a partner.

☞ Remember!!

Anyone can be a victim of dating violence. Both boys and girls are victims, but boys and girls abuse their partners in different ways. Girls are more likely to yell, threaten to hurt themselves, pinch, slap, scratch, or kick. Boys injure girls more and are more likely to punch their partner and force them to participate in unwanted sexual activity. Some teen victims experience violence occasionally. Others are abused more often, sometimes daily.

- 50–80% of teens have reported knowing others who were involved in violent relationships.

- Teens identifying as gay, lesbian, and bisexual are as likely to experience violence in same-sex dating relationships as youths involved in opposite sex dating.

- Many studies indicate that, as a dating relationship becomes more serious, the potential for, and nature of, violent behavior escalates.

- Young women, ages 16 to 24 years, experience the highest rates of relationship violence.

Get Help

- If you think you are in an abusive relationship, get help immediately. Don't keep your concerns to yourself.

- Talk to someone you trust like a parent, teacher, school principal, counselor, or nurse.

- If you choose to tell, you should know that some adults are mandated reporters. This means they are legally required to report neglect or abuse to someone else, such as the police or child protective services. You can ask people if they are mandated reporters and then decide what you want to do. Some examples of mandated reporters are teachers, counselors, doctors, social workers, and in some cases, even coaches or activity leaders. If you want help deciding whom to talk to, call the National Crime Victim Helpline at 1-800-FYI-CALL or an anonymous crisis line in your area. You might also want to talk to a trusted family member, a friend's parent, an adult neighbor or friend, an older sibling or cousin, or other experienced person who you trust.

Help Yourself

Think about ways you can be safer. This means thinking about what to do, where to go for help, and who to call ahead of time.

- Where can you go for help?
- Who can you call?

- Who will help you?

- How will you escape a violent situation?

Here are other precautions you can take.

- Let friends or family know when you are afraid or need help.

- When you go out, say where you are going and when you'll be back.

- In an emergency, call 911 or your local police department.

- Memorize important phone numbers, such as the people to contact or places to go in an emergency.

- Keep spare change, calling cards, or a cell phone handy for immediate access to communication.

- Go out in a group or with other couples.

- Have money available for transportation if you need to take a taxi, bus, or subway to escape.

Help Someone Else

If you know someone who might be in an abusive relationship, you can help.

- Tell the person that you are worried.

- Be a good listener.

- Offer your friendship and support.

- Ask how you can help.

- Encourage your friend to seek help.

- Educate yourself about dating violence and healthy relationships.

- Avoid any confrontations with the abuser. This could be dangerous for you and your friend.

☞ Remember!!
Being a victim of dating violence is not your fault. Nothing you say, wear, or do gives anyone the right to hurt you.

Chapter 22

Physical Fighting Among Teenagers

Introduction

Is physical fighting among teenagers a serious problem in the United States?

Physical fights typically involve two or more teens that have chosen to use physical force to resolve a conflict or argument.

Because physical fights are so common, many people dismiss them as a normal part of growing up. While it is true that teens (and teenage boys in particular) have always engaged in fistfights, today, many teens carry deadly weapons. Fights that involve weapons, such as guns, knives, and clubs, are a major cause of serious injuries and death among teenagers.

Why do some teens fight?

When junior and senior high students around the nation were asked to identify the causes of the most recent fights they had witnessed, most frequent responses were the following:

- Someone insulted someone else or treated them disrespectfully (54 percent).

About This Chapter: Information in this chapter is from "Physical Fighting Among Teenagers," National Youth Violence Prevention Resource Center, 2002.

- There was an ongoing feud or disagreement (44 percent).

- Someone was hit, pushed, shoved, or bumped (42 percent).

- Someone spread rumors or said things about someone else (40 percent).

- Someone could not control his or her anger (39 percent).

> ♣ **It's A Fact!!**
>
> Increasing numbers of teenagers are learning that while disagreements are inevitable, there are more effective ways to resolve conflicts and keep the peace.

- Other people were watching or encouraging the fight (34 percent).

- Someone who likes to fight a lot was involved (26 percent).

- Someone did not want to look like a loser (21 percent).

- There was an argument over a boyfriend or girlfriend (19 percent).

- Someone wanted to keep a reputation or get a name (17 percent).

Are some teens more likely to get into fights than others?

- **Male teens are much more likely to fight than females.** In a recent national survey, 44 percent of male high school students versus 27 percent of female students said they had been in a fight in the past year.

- **Younger teens are much more likely to fight than older teens.** In a recent national survey, over 40 percent of 9th graders said they had been in a fight in the past year, in contrast with only 30 percent of 12th graders.

- **Teens who use alcohol and drugs, such as marijuana, cocaine, and anabolic steroids, are much more likely to fight.** In addition, fight participants who are drunk or high are much more likely to use weapons and cause serious injuries. One study found that when the participants were drunk or high, over 60 percent were seriously injured (with broken bones, loss of consciousness, knife or gunshot wound), and over half used weapons. In contrast, when alcohol and drugs were not involved, only 18 percent of the fights involved serious injuries or weapon use.

- **Teens who carry weapons are more likely to be involved in physical fights.** One study found that students who had carried weapons were more than twice as likely to get in fights. Another found that the students who had fought the most at school were almost ten times more likely to have carried a gun to school in the past month than those students who did not fight. Teens who carry weapons are also more likely to suffer serious injuries.

Do teens who fight put themselves at risk in other ways?

Over half of the teens that fight also participate in behaviors that can put them or those around them at risk for harm. Such behaviors include using illegal drugs, binge drinking, carrying weapons, and having unsafe sex.

One national survey found that of the youth who reported fighting in the past month:

- 45 percent had unsafe sex in the last 3 months;
- 41 percent had two or more sex partners in the last 3 months;
- 39 percent had driven a car while drunk or high in the last month;
- 26 percent had carried a gun in the last month;
- 24 percent had attempted suicide during the past 12 months; and
- 13 percent had used cocaine in the last month.

Why do some teens believe fighting is a solution to conflict?

Teens who are frequently involved in fights often don't know how to control their anger and prevent or avoid conflicts. They often believe that fighting is the only acceptable solution.

♣ It's A Fact!!
When teens fight, those who carry handguns are three times more likely to require medical attention than those who do not carry weapons.

For example, students who fight at school are much less likely than other students to believe that it is effective to apologize or avoid or walk away from someone who wants to fight. They are also more likely to believe their families would want them to hit back if someone hit them first.

Students who have trouble controlling their anger or who are predisposed toward fighting (agreeing with statements such as, "If I am challenged,
I am going to fight," or "Avoiding fights is a sign of weakness") are at least 50
percent more likely to get in fights.

What You Can Do

Helping Yourself

Learn about ways to resolve arguments and fights peacefully and encourage your friends to do the same. Many schools, churches, and after-school
programs offer training in conflict resolution skills. In the meantime, you
can to the following:

- Figure out what methods work for you to control your anger (like
  leaving a tense situation temporarily or finding a calm person to talk
  to) and use them before losing control.

- Before a fight, think about what the consequences of different actions
  will be—anger and violence versus walking away from a dispute or
  compromise.

- Do not carry a gun or other weapons. Weapons escalate conflicts and
  increase the chances that you will be seriously harmed or that you will
  accidentally harm someone else. It is also illegal for a teen to carry a
  handgun, and it can lead to criminal charges and arrest.

- Never fight with anyone using drugs or alcohol or likely to have a weapon.

- When in a conflict, try to think of solutions that will give both sides
  something and try to understand your opponent's point of view. Show
  respect for your opponent's rights and position.

- Decide on your options for handling the problem such as talking the
  problem out calmly with the people involved, avoiding the problem by
  staying away from certain people, or diffusing the problem by resolving to take it less seriously. Try to use humor to cool hostility.

- If you feel intensely angry, fearful, or anxious, talk about it with an
  adult you trust.

If someone is threatening you and you feel that you are in serious danger, do not take matters into your own hands. Find an adult you can trust and discuss your fears or contact school administrators or the police. Take precautions for your safety such as avoiding being alone and staying with a group of friends if possible.

Helping Your Community

Lead by example. Never physically or verbally harm, bully, tease, or intimidate others.

Be a "positive bystander." When you see a fight starting, do not watch or egg others on to fight. When a fight has bystanders cheering it on, it is generally more dangerous, with more serious injuries. Whenever possible, try to promote a peaceful resolution.

Get involved. Become an active partner in violence prevention efforts in your school and community. Work with your school to create a process for students to safely report threats, intimidation, weapon possession, drug selling, gang activity, and vandalism. Become an advocate for programs such as mentoring, conflict resolution, peer assistance leadership, teen courts, or anger management.

Work with others. Help develop and participate in activities to promote understanding and respecting differences.

Mentor other students. Volunteer to be a mentor for younger students and/or provide tutoring for your peers. Those who have positive role models often are steered away from a path of violence in their lives and learn to resolve problems peacefully.

Chapter 23

Bullying

In the United States, bullying among children and teenagers has often been dismissed as a normal part of growing up. Little attention has been paid to the devastating effects of bullying or to the connection between bullying and other forms of violence. In recent years, however, students and adults around the country have begun to make a commitment to stop bullying in their schools and communities.

What is bullying?

Bullying includes a wide variety of behaviors, but all involve a person or a group repeatedly trying to harm someone who is weaker or more vulnerable. It can involve direct attacks (such as hitting, threatening or intimidating, maliciously teasing and taunting, name-calling, making sexual remarks, and stealing or damaging belongings) or subtler, indirect attacks (such as spreading rumors or encouraging others to reject or exclude someone).

How common is bullying?

Almost 30 percent of teens in the United States (or over 5.7 million) are estimated to be involved in bullying as either a bully, a target of bullying, or both. In a recent national survey of students in grades six to ten, 13 percent

About This Chapter: Information in this chapter is from "Bullying," National Youth Violence Prevention Resource Center, 2002.

reported bullying others, 11 percent reported being the target of bullies, and another 6 percent said they bullied others and were bullied themselves.

Bullying occurs more frequently among boys than girls. Teenage boys are much more likely to bully others and to be the targets of bullies. While both boys and girls say others bully them by making fun of the way they look or talk, boys are more likely to report being hit, slapped, or pushed. Teenage girls are more often the targets of rumors and sexual comments. While teenage boys target both boys and girls, teenage girls most often bully other girls, using more subtle and indirect forms of aggression than boys. For example, instead of physically harming others, they are more likely to spread gossip or encourage others to reject or exclude another girl.

How does bullying affect teens that are the targets of bullies?

Bullying can lead teenagers to feel tense, anxious, and afraid. It can affect their concentration in school and can lead them to avoid school in some cases. If bullying continues for some time, it can begin to affect teens' self-esteem and feelings of self-worth. It also can increase their social isolation, leading them to become withdrawn and depressed, anxious and insecure. In extreme cases, bullying can be devastating for teens, with long-term consequences. Some teens feel compelled to take drastic measures such as carrying weapons for protection or seeking violent revenge. Others, in desperation, even consider suicide.

❖ **It's A Fact!!**
Limited available data suggest that bullying is much more common among younger teens than older teens. As teens grow older, they are less likely to bully others and to be the targets of bullies.

Source: National Youth Violence Prevention Resource Center, 2002.

How can bullying affect those teens that witness the bullying?

In one study of junior high and high school students, over 88 percent said they had witnessed bullying in their schools. Teens who witness bullying can feel guilty or helpless for not standing up to a bully on behalf of a classmate or friend or for not reporting the incident to someone who could help. They may

✤ It's A Fact!!

Researchers have found that years later, long after the bullying has stopped, adults who were bullied as teens have higher levels of depression and poorer self-esteem than other adults.

Source: National Youth Violence Prevention Resource Center, 2002.

experience even greater guilt if they are drawn into bullying by pressure from their peers. Some teens deal with these feelings of guilt by blaming the victim and deciding that he or she deserved the abuse. Teens sometimes also feel compelled to end a friendship or avoid being seen with the bullied teen to avoid losing status or being targeted themselves.

Which teens are most likely to become bullies?

While many people believe bullies act tough in order to hide feelings of insecurity and self-loathing, in fact, bullies tend to be confident with high self-esteem. They are generally physically aggressive, with pro-violence attitudes, and are typically hot-tempered, easily angered, and impulsive, with a low tolerance for frustration. Bullies have a strong need to dominate others and usually have little empathy for their targets. Male bullies are often physically bigger and stronger than their peers. Bullies tend to get in trouble more often, and to dislike and do more poorly in school, than teens that do not bully others. They are also more likely to fight, drink, and smoke than their peers.

Teens who come from homes where parents provide little emotional support for their children, fail to monitor their activities, or have little involvement in their lives, are at greater risk for engaging in bullying behavior. Parents' discipline styles are also related to bullying behavior. An extremely permissive or excessively harsh approach to discipline can increase the risk of teenage bullying.

Surprisingly, bullies appear to have little difficulty in making friends. Their friends typically share their pro-violence attitudes and problem behaviors (such as drinking and smoking) and may be involved in bullying as well. These friends are often followers who do not initiate bullying, but participate in it.

As mentioned above, some teenagers not only bully others but are also the targets of bullies themselves. Like other bullies, they tend to do poorly in school and engage in a number of problem behaviors. They also tend to be socially isolated with few friends and poor relationships with their classmates.

What can schools do to stop bullying?

Effective programs have been developed to reduce bullying in schools. Research has found that bullying is most likely to occur in schools where there is a lack of adult supervision during breaks, where teachers and students are indifferent to or accept bullying behavior, and where rules against bullying are not consistently enforced.

> **✣ It's A Fact!!**
> **What are the long-term consequences of bullying behavior?**
>
> Bullying is often a warning sign that children and teens are heading for trouble and are at risk for serious violence. Teens (particularly boys) who bully are more likely to engage in other anti-social/delinquent behavior (e.g., vandalism, shoplifting, truancy, and drug use) into adulthood. They are four times more likely than nonbullies to be convicted of crimes by age 24 with 60 percent of bullies having at least one criminal conviction.
>
> Source: National Youth Violence Prevention Resource Center, 2002.

While approaches that simply crack down on individual bullies are seldom effective, when there is a school-wide commitment to end bullying, it can be reduced by up to 50 percent. One effective approach focuses on changing school and classroom climates by raising awareness about bullying, increasing teacher and parent involvement and supervision, forming clear rules and strong social norms against bullying, and providing support and protection for all students. This approach involves teachers, principals, students, and everyone associated with the school including janitors, cafeteria workers, and crossing guards. Adults become aware of the extent of bullying at the school, and they involve themselves in changing the situation, rather than looking the other way. Students pledge not to bully other students, to help students who are bullied, and to make a point to include students who are left out.

What can you do if you are being bullied?

Talk to your parents or an adult you can trust such as a teacher, school counselor, or principal. Many teens that are targets of bullies do not talk to adults because they feel embarrassed, ashamed, or fearful, and they believe they should be able to handle the problem on their own. Others believe that involving adults will only make the situation worse. While in some cases it is possible to end bullying without adult intervention, in other more extreme cases, it is necessary to involve school officials and even law enforcement. Talk to a trusted adult who can help you develop a plan to end the bullying and provide you with the support you need. If the first adult you approach is not receptive, find another adult who will support and help you.

It is not useful to blame yourself for a bully's actions. You can do a few things, however, that may help if a bully begins to harass you. Do not retaliate against a bully or let the bully see how much he or she has upset you. If bullies know they are getting to you, they are likely to torment you more. If at all possible, stay calm and respond evenly and firmly or else say nothing and walk away. Sometimes you can make a joke, laugh at yourself, and use humor to defuse a situation.

Act confident. Hold your head up, stand up straight, make eye contact, and walk confidently. A bully will be less likely to single you out if you project self-confidence.

Try to make friends with other students. A bully is more likely to leave you alone if you are with your friends. This is especially true if you and your friends stick up for each other.

Avoid situations where bullying can happen. If at all possible, avoid being alone with bullies. If bullying occurs on the way to or from school, you may want to take a different route, leave at a different time, or find others to walk to and from school with. If bullying occurs at school, avoid areas that are isolated or unsupervised by adults, and stick with friends as much as possible.

If necessary, take steps to rebuild your self-confidence. Bullying can affect your self-confidence and belief in yourself. Finding activities you enjoy

♣ It's A Fact!!
What is cyber bullying?

Cyber bullying is repeatedly hurting someone else through the use of technology. So, instead of whispering a rumor to a friend, a bully might e-mail or instant message that rumor or post it on the internet for everyone to see; or the bully might use technology to ignore you. An example of this would be a friend all of a sudden ignoring your e-mails or instant messages.

Types of cyber bullying include the following:

• blogs

• instant messaging

• e-mail

• chat rooms

• text messaging

Many teens today, especially girls, use technology to bully others. In fact, one study found that twice as many girls as boys had bullied someone online.

Here are some tips that may help protect you from cyber-bullying:

• Do not give out personal information online, whether in instant message profiles, chat rooms, blogs, or on websites.

• Do not tell anyone your e-mail or instant messaging passwords, even your friends.

• If someone sends a mean or threatening message, do not respond. Save it and show it to a trusted adult.

• Do not be a cyber bully because you just may find yourself on the other end of the cyber bullying down the road.

Source: GirlsHealth.gov, sponsored by the National Women's Health Information Center, U.S. Department of Health and Human Services, September 2006.

and are good at can help to restore your self-esteem. Take time to explore new interests and develop new talents and skills. Bullying can also leave you feeling rejected, isolated, and alone. It is important to try to make new friendships with people who share your interests. Consider participating in extra-curricular activities or joining a group outside of school such as an after-school program, church youth group, or sports team.

Do not resort to violence or carry a gun or other weapon. Carrying a gun will not make you safer. Guns often escalate conflicts and increase the chances you will be seriously harmed. You also run the risk that the gun may be turned on you or an innocent person will be hurt. And you may do something in a moment of fear or anger you will regret for the rest of your life. Finally, it is illegal for a teen to carry a handgun; it can lead to criminal charges and arrest.

What can you do if someone else is being bullied?

Refuse to join in if you see someone being bullied. It can be hard to resist if a bully tries to get you to taunt or torment someone, and you may fear the bully will turn on you if you do not participate, but try to stand firm.

Attempt to defuse bullying situations when you see them starting up. For example, try to draw attention away from the targeted person or take the bully aside and ask him/her to "cool it." Do not place yourself at risk, however.

If you can do so without risk to your own safety, get a teacher, parent, or other responsible adult to come help immediately.

Speak up and/or offer support to bullied teens when you witness bullying. For example, help them up if they have been tripped or knocked down. If you feel you cannot do this at the time, privately support those being hurt with words of kindness or condolence later.

Encourage the bullied teen to talk with parents or a trusted adult. Offer to go with the person if it would help. Tell an adult yourself if the teen is unwilling to report the bullying. If necessary for your safety, do this anonymously.

Chapter 24

Hazing

Hazing Defined

Hazing refers to any activity expected of someone joining a group (or to maintain full status in a group) that humiliates, degrades, or risks emotional and/or physical harm, regardless of the person's willingness to participate. In years past, hazing practices were typically considered harmless pranks or comical antics associated with young men in college fraternities.

Today we know that hazing extends far beyond college fraternities and is experienced by boys/men and girls/women in school groups, university organizations, athletic teams, the military, and other social and professional organizations. Hazing is a complex social problem that is shaped by power dynamics operating in a group and/or organization and within a particular cultural context.

Hazing activities are generally considered to be physically abusive, hazardous, and/or sexually violating. The specific behaviors or activities within these categories vary widely among participants, groups, and settings. While alcohol use is common in many types of hazing, other examples of typical hazing practices include personal servitude; sleep deprivation and restrictions on personal

About This Chapter: This chapter includes text from "Hazing Defined," "High School Hazing," and "Hazing and Athletics," Copyright © StopHazing.org, www.stophazing.org; accessed March 2007.

hygiene; yelling, swearing, and insulting new members/rookies; being forced to wear embarrassing or humiliating attire in public; consumption of vile substances or smearing of such on one's skin; brandings; physical beatings; binge drinking and drinking games; sexual simulation and sexual assault.

High School Hazing

Frequent misconceptions about hazing include the idea that hazing is nothing more than harmless pranks and that it is a practice largely isolated to college fraternities. The reality is that hazing activities occur in many different arenas. As a recent study indicates, hazing takes place in both men's and women's organizations and is common among student groups in middle/high schools—particularly athletic teams. To date, there has been no large-scale research focused solely on hazing at the high school level.

Hazing at any age can be exceedingly harmful. Hazing at the high school level is particularly troubling because the developmental stages of adolescence create a situation in which many students are more vulnerable to peer pressure due to the tremendous need for belonging, making friends, and finding approval in one's peer group. Further, the danger of hazing at the high school level is heightened by the lack of awareness and policy development/enforcement around this issue. While many colleges and universities in the U.S. have instituted anti-hazing policies and educational awareness programs related to hazing, very few secondary schools have done the same.

A major part of the problem is the lack of understanding among the general population about hazing. Hazing practices in high schools are often overlooked and dismissed as mere "traditions" because students, parents, teachers, coaches, and administrators do not understand the definition of hazing and how it operates in society. Many who are aware of hazing activities do not concern themselves with confronting

❖ It's A Fact!!
Hazing is a form of abuse and victimization. This is why it is crucial to promote anti-hazing education and support for victims at the middle and high school levels.

Source: From "High School Hazing," © StopHazing.org.

the behavior because of the popular myths and misconceptions that are attached to the term. Hazing is not about harmless traditions or silly antics—hazing is about abuse of power and violation of human dignity.

Hazing And Athletics

Although hazing has often been thought to exist primarily in fraternities and sororities, a 1999 study by Alfred University and the National Collegiate Athletic Association (NCAA) found that approximately 80% of college athletes had been subjected to some form of hazing. Half were required to participate in drinking contests or alcohol related initiations, while two thirds were subjected to humiliating hazing. Additionally, much of the reported hazing in high schools occurs during initiations related to athletic teams with many problems arising during pre-season sports camps. Some of the recent high profile hazing incidents in the news have involved brutal initiations in high school sports. Hazing also occurs among professional sports teams as documented in numerous news media accounts.

Despite widespread reports of hazing in sport, many coaches and athletic directors did not identify hazing as a problem on their teams (according to the Alfred/NCAA study). However, many educational institutions and associations are seriously addressing the problem of hazing and athletes.

Much education is still needed to eliminate harmful hazing in athletics. Something on which most educators, coaches, and advocates agree is the best way to end hazing is to begin by sending a clear anti-hazing message. Then implement a strong anti-hazing policy, communicate it clearly, and enforce it when incidents occur.

Has gang violence become increasingly deadly over the last few decades?

Yes. Some people have blamed this change on gangs' growing participation in the drug trade and "drug wars". That does not appear to be the primary reason for the dramatic increase in gang violence and homicides, however. Instead, researchers believe that gang violence has become more dangerous because of the increasing availability of more lethal weapons and the growing use of cars in drive-by attacks on other gangs.

> ♣ **It's A Fact!!**
> Joining a gang is dangerous. Violent conflict between gangs is common, and gang members are at least 60 times more likely to be killed than the rest of the population.

Is gang membership on the rise?

There has been a dramatic increase in gang activity in the United States since the 1970s. In the 1970s, gangs were active in less than half the states, but now every state reports youth gang activity; and, while many people think of gangs as just an inner-city problem, that is clearly no longer the case. In the past few decades, we have seen a dramatic increase in the growth of gang problems in smaller cities, towns, and rural areas.

Since 1996, the overall number of gangs and gang members in the United States has decreased. However, in cities with a population over 25,000, gang involvement still remains near peak levels.

How old are most gang members?

Although some gang members are as young as 12, the average age is about 17 to 18 years. Not many people realize that around half of youth gang members are 18 or older. These older members are much more likely to be involved in serious and violent crimes than younger members. Only about one in four gang members are ages 15 to 17.

For most teens, gang membership is a brief phase. One-half to two-thirds of teen gang members leave the gang by the end of their first year.

Do many girls join gangs?

Male teens are much more likely to join gangs than female teens. Police reports indicate that only about 6% of gang members are female and that 39% of gangs have some female members. These estimates are probably low, however. One 11-city survey of eighth-graders found that 38% of gang members were female.

Female gang members are less likely to be involved in criminal behavior than males, but they are still an important concern. In one survey, 78% of female gang members reported being involved in gang fights, 65% reported carrying a weapon for protection, and 39% reported attacking someone with a weapon.

What can you do?

Find positive ways to spend your time and energy. Many teens join gangs because they are bored, lacking in purpose, or looking for a way to belong; but there are other options. Sports, recreational, and after-school programs give you a great chance to meet new people, explore new interests, develop new talents and skills, and to connect with people that really care about you and your well-being.

Stay away from gangs and gang members. Be aware of clothing, colors, and symbols used by gangs in your area, and avoid them. If you look like a gang member or are seen with a gang member, other gangs may mistake you for a real gang member. You have a very good chance of being the innocent target of violent gang behavior.

Do not carry a gun or other weapons. Carrying a gun is not likely to make you safer. Guns often escalate conflicts and increase the chances that you will be seriously harmed. If someone is threatening you and you feel that you are

> ♣ **It's A Fact!!**
> **Why do teens join gangs?**
>
> Teens join gangs for a variety of reasons. Some are seeking excitement; others are looking for prestige, protection, a chance to make money, or a sense of belonging. Few teens are forced to join gangs; in most cases, teens can refuse to join without fear of retaliation.

fear, vulnerability, insecurity, distrust, and outrage. They can also launch cycles of retaliation and counter-retaliation among groups.

Most hate crimes are committed by and against teens and young adults.

Almost two-thirds of reported attacks are committed by individuals under the age of 24. Although people of all racial and ethnic groups commit hate crimes, young white males commit most of them.

Most victims of violent hate crimes are also young. More than half of the victims of reported hate violence are age 24 or under, and nearly a third are under 18. African Americans, Jews, Arab Americans and Muslims, new immigrants, lesbians, gay men, and women are some of the most frequently targeted groups.

Why do teens and young adults commit hate crimes?

The majority of people who commit hate crimes are not members of organized hate groups, although they may be influenced by their propaganda. Instead, they are individuals who believe negative stereotypes about groups and act on impulse. Their prejudice blinds them to the immorality of what they are doing.

♣ **It's A Fact!!**
Prejudice is at the heart of all hate crimes. Although most prejudiced individuals do not commit hate crimes, prejudice is a key motivation for those who do.

The majority are "thrill seekers" who randomly target members of minority groups for harassment and violence. They often do this out of boredom and are seeking some excitement. They may also be trying to impress their peers or prove their toughness.

Others feel that members of a group are a threat to their way of life, neighborhood, place of work, or economic well-being, and hence attack them. Their violence is meant to send a message and to spread fear and intimidation among all members of the group.

A very small percentage of people who commit hate crimes believe that they are on a mission to rid the world of some perceived evil. These individuals are often psychotic, suffering from a mental illness.

What You Can Do

Teenagers and young adults can play an important role in reducing and preventing hate violence. Consider some of the following suggestions:

- **Start with yourself.** Try to broaden your social circle to include others who are different from you. Be mindful of your language, avoid stereotypical remarks, and challenge those made by others. Speak out against jokes and slurs that target people or groups. Silence sends a message that you are in agreement. It is not enough to refuse to laugh.

- **Read books about diverse cultures, traditions, and lifestyles in our society.** Learning about others' cultures and traditions can help you be more compassionate and understanding. It can also help you better understand points of view that are different from your own.

- **Talk with your friends, parents, and school staff about how you and your classmates can respond to hateful attitudes and behaviors.** Newspapers, magazines, movies, and television shows that you have seen on these subjects can be great ways to start a discussion about hate crimes and intolerance.

- **Research and find out about hate crimes that have occurred in your community and what was done to respond to them.** Identify any hate groups active in your community, then share the information by publishing an article in a school or local newspaper or talking to community groups or groups of students.

- **Join an existing group that is promoting tolerance in your school or community, or launch your own effort.** Join with other students to create anti-hate policies and programs in your school. Coordinate an event that brings diverse people and groups together. Find ways to show support and solidarity for groups when one of their members is a victim of hate violence.

> **♣ It's A Fact!!**
> None of us are born hating people who are different from us. These attitudes are learned from parents, schools, peers, the media, and society in general. So it is possible for all of us to learn to appreciate, respect, and celebrate our differences.

Chapter 27

School Violence And Effects Of School Violence Exposure

School Violence

In the last few years, a great deal of media attention has been focused on school shootings. This has led many teens to become concerned about their own safety, wondering whether such tragic violence could happen in their schools.

However, in terms of risk for homicide, schools are about the safest place for teens—safer than their homes or their neighborhoods—and violent deaths at schools or school events are extremely rare.

Less than 1% of the murders of children and teens in the United States are school-related, and there is no evidence that school-related homicides are on the rise. You are much more likely to be struck by lightening than to be killed at your school.

This is not to suggest that school violence is not a serious problem in the United States.

About This Chapter: This chapter begins with text excerpted from "School Violence," National Youth Violence Prevention Resource Center, 2002. It continues with text from "School-Associated Violent Deaths," National Center for Injury Prevention and Control, Centers for Disease Control and Prevention, October 2006.

Although incidents like the one in Littleton, Colorado, tend to get all the attention, if you have ever been ruthlessly teased, laughed at, shoved around, or bullied at school, you know there is more to violence in school than mass shootings.

In fact, school violence includes a range of activities including bullying, threatening remarks, physical fights, assaults with or without weapons, and gang violence.

What You Can Do

Start with yourself. Make a commitment not to contribute to violence in any way. Do not bully, tease, or spread negative gossip about others. Respect others and value differences. Try to broaden your social circle to include others who are different from you.

Learn about ways to resolve arguments and fights without violence, and encourage your friends to do the same. Many schools, churches, and after-school programs offer training in conflict resolution skills.

Do not carry a gun. Teens sometimes carry guns because they are afraid, but carrying a gun will not make you safer.

Guns often escalate conflicts and increase the chances that you will be seriously harmed. You also run the risk that the gun may be turned on you or that an innocent person will be hurt, and you may do something in a moment of fear or anger that you will regret for the rest of your life.

Finally, it is illegal for a teen to carry a handgun, and it can lead to criminal charges and arrest.

✔ Quick Tip

If you know someone is carrying a gun or planning to harm someone else, report him or her. Most of us have learned from an early age that it is wrong to tattle, but in some instances it is the most courageous thing you can do. Tell a trusted adult, such as a teacher, guidance counselor, principal, or parent. If you are afraid and believe that telling will put you in danger or lead to retaliation, find a way to anonymously contact the authorities.

Source: National Youth Violence Prevention Resource Center, 2002.

How can you protect yourself without a gun? If someone is threatening you, and you feel that you are in serious danger, do not take matters into your own hands. Find an adult you can trust and discuss your fears or contact school administrators or the police. Take precautions for your safety such as avoiding being alone and staying with a group of friends if possible.

Take the initiative to make your school safer. Join an existing group that is promoting nonviolence at your school, or launch your own effort. You might want to consider some of the following ideas:

• Start a conflict resolution program to teach students to handle conflict peacefully.

• Start a drama troupe to develop productions with nonviolence themes such as peaceful conflict resolution, respect for diversity, and tolerance.

• Launch a school crime watch program.

• Plan a nonviolence rally or dance, and encourage other students to make a commitment to avoiding conflicts.

• Start a "peace pledge" campaign, in which students promise to settle disagreements without violence, to reject weapons, and to work toward a safe school for all.

• Set up an anonymous hot line so students can share their concerns if they feel threatened or know of someone who may become violent.

• Set up a forum for students to talk about how school violence is affecting their lives and to brainstorm about possible solutions.

School-Associated Violent Deaths

To learn how school shootings may be prevented, the Centers for Disease Control and Prevention (CDC) is conducting ongoing research to learn more about the nature of school-associated violent deaths. Here are some of the key facts from this research:

• The number of children and youth homicides that are school-related make up one percent of the total number of child and youth homicides in the United States.

♣ It's A Fact!!

Exposure to violence generates a sense of fear and leads to acts intended to reduce or control fear.

Exposure to violence is psychologically toxic. This exposure may produce the following:

- generalized emotional distress
- disruptions in interpersonal relationships
- problems with aggression, conduct disorder, and truancy
- cognitive, psychological, and physical issues related to learning and teaching
- physical symptoms such as chronic fatigue

The effects of exposure to violence in schools may spread to others within the school setting. This spread, or "contagion," changes the school setting in ways that negatively alter school interactions and interfere with the schools' capacity to achieve its educational and social goals.

Widespread concern about violence within a school may reduce the quality of teaching, disrupt classroom discipline, limit teachers' availability to students before or after the school day, and reduce students' motivation to attend school and/or willingness to participate in extracurricular activities.

Source: From "Exposure to Urban Violence," a fact sheet from the Center for the Study and Prevention of Violence, University of Colorado at Boulder. © 1998 University of Colorado. Reprinted with permission.

- Most school-associated violent deaths occurred during transition times such as the start or end of the school day or during the lunch period.

- We have also seen that school-associated homicides are more likely to occur at the start of each semester.

- Nearly 50 percent of the homicide perpetrators (this includes adults, children, and youth) gave some type of warning signal (e.g., a threat, a note) prior to the event.

- Among the students who committed a school-associated homicide, 20% were known to have been victims of bullying, and 12% were known to have expressed suicidal thoughts or engage in suicidal behavior.

Preventive Measures That May Help Prevent School-Associated Violent Deaths

CDC in partnership with the Departments of Education and Justice is gathering information about school-associated violent deaths to identify trends that can help schools develop preventive measures to protect and promote the health, safety, and development of all students. These prevention measures include the following:

- Encouraging efforts to reduce crowding, increase supervision, and institute plans/policies to handle disputes during transition times that may reduce the likelihood of potential conflicts and injuries.

- Taking threats seriously. Students need to know who to go to when they have learned of a threat to anyone at the school, while parents, educators, and mentors should be encouraged to take an active role in helping troubled children and teens.

- Taking talk of suicide seriously. It is important to address risk factors for suicidal behavior when trying to prevent violence toward self and others.

- Promoting prevention programs that are designed to help teachers and other school staff recognize and respond to incidences of bullying between students.

- Ensuring at the start of each semester that schools' security plans are being enforced and that staff are trained and prepared to use the plans.

- Homicides, followed by suicides and isolated suicides, account for nearly one in five of the violent deaths.

☞ Remember!!

School shootings are sobering and tragic events that cause much concern about the safety of children. Despite these events, schools remain a very safe place for children to spend their days. In fact, the vast majority of children and youth homicides occur outside school hours and property.

Source: Centers for Disease Control and Prevention, October 2006.

Chapter 28

Teen Firearm Violence

Facts About Teen Firearm Violence

During the late 1980s and early 1990s, teen gun violence increased dramatically in the United States. More and more teens began to acquire and carry guns, leading to a sharp increase in gun deaths and injuries.

In recent years, however, it appears that the tide has begun to turn. Fewer teens are carrying guns now, and gun-related murders and suicides have begun to decline. Even so, many teens still illegally carry guns and harm others and themselves.

Access To Guns

Federal law makes it illegal for anyone under the age of 18 to have a handgun, yet teens have little difficulty in getting them. Some get guns from their friends, while others borrow, buy, or steal them.

Many teens have access to guns in their homes. A recent study found that 43% of households in the U.S. with children and teens had at least one gun. More than 1 in 5 gun owners with children under 18 said that they stored their weapons loaded, and about 1 in 11 said that their weapons were stored loaded and unlocked. Another study found that parents owned the guns used in more than half of the teen suicides and suicide attempts.

About This Chapter: Information in this chapter is from "Teen Firearm Violence," National Youth Violence Prevention Resource Center, 2002.

Gun Carrying And Use

Many teens are carrying guns today, although the numbers have decreased in recent years. Male teens, in particular, are likely to possess and carry guns.

Gun Suicide

Guns are the number one way that teens take their own lives. Almost 60% of teen suicide deaths in recent years have involved guns.

♣ **It's A Fact!!**
The Federal Bureau of Investigation's *Crime in the United States* estimated that 66% of the 16,137 murders in 2004 were committed with firearms.

Source: Excerpted from "Firearms and Crime Statistics," Bureau of Justice Statistics, Office of Justice Programs, U.S. Department of Justice, September 2006.

When teens shoot themselves, they most often do so in their own homes. Teens are at a far greater risk for suicide when there are loaded and accessible guns at home.

Gun Homicide And Assault

Along with the increase in the number of teens carrying guns in the late 1980s and early 1990s came a sharp increase in teen gun-related homicides. The increase in gun carrying meant that arguments once settled by fistfights were settled with guns.

For every person killed with a gun, another three people are treated in hospital emergency rooms for non-accidental gun injuries.

What You Can Do

Do not carry a gun. Teens sometimes carry guns because they are afraid or because they want to intimidate others, but carrying a gun will not make you safer.

Guns escalate conflicts and increase the chances that you will be seriously harmed. If you carry a gun, you are twice as likely to become the victim of gun violence. You also run the risk that the gun may be turned on you or that an innocent person will be hurt, and, you may do something in a moment of fear or anger that you will regret for the rest of your life.

Finally, it is illegal for a teen to carry a handgun, and it can lead to criminal charges and arrest.

How can you protect yourself without a gun? Learn about ways to resolve arguments and fights without guns or violence, and encourage your friends to do the same. Many schools, churches, and after-school programs offer training in conflict resolution skills.

If someone is threatening you, and you feel that you are in serious danger, do not take matters into your own hands. Find an adult you can trust and discuss your fears, or contact school administrators or the police. Take precautions for your safety such as avoiding being alone and staying with a group of friends if possible.

If you know someone is carrying a gun, report him or her. Most of us have learned from an early age that it is wrong to "snitch" on someone else, but in some instances, it is the most courageous thing you can do. Tell a trusted adult such as a teacher, guidance counselor, principal, or parent. If you are afraid and believe that telling will put you in danger or lead to retaliation, find a way to anonymously contact the authorities.

If your parents have a gun at home, give them the facts. Let them know that the number one way teens commit suicide is by firearms; and let them know how often children and teens are injured, or die, after they get their hands on a gun they find at home.

If your parents choose to keep a gun at home, encourage them to empty the bullets and to lock the gun and bullets in separate places.

If your parents do lock up guns, tell them if you know how to access the guns and suggest that they find a different location for the guns and/or keys. Why? Because if you know where keys are kept, it is likely that others, such as younger brothers and sisters, may also know.

Your local police can provide your parents with information about safe storage and gun locks.

Make sure you steer clear of guns in your friends' homes, and encourage them to do the same. Stay away from teens that are attracted to guns and see them as symbols of power, not realizing how dangerous they are.

Chapter 29

Terrorism

General Information About Terrorism

Terrorism is the use of force or violence against persons or property in violation of the criminal laws of the United States for purposes of intimidation, coercion, or ransom.

Terrorists often use threats to do the following:

• Create fear among the public.

• Try to convince citizens that their government is powerless to prevent terrorism.

• Get immediate publicity for their causes.

High-risk targets for acts of terrorism include military and civilian government facilities, international airports, large cities, and high-profile landmarks. Terrorists might also target large public gatherings, water and food supplies, utilities, and corporate centers. Further, terrorists are capable of

About This Chapter: Information in this chapter is from the following documents produced by Federal Emergency Management Agency (www.fema.gov), U.S. Department of Homeland Security: "General Information About Terrorism," April 2006, "Explosions," April 2006, "Bomb Threat," March 2006, "During an Explosion," March 2006, "Suspicious Packages and Letters," March 2006, "Biological Threats," March 2006, "During a Biological Attack," March 2006, "Chemical Threats," March 2006, and "During a Chemical Attack," March 2006.

spreading fear by sending explosives or chemical and biological agents through the mail.

Within the immediate area of a terrorist event, you would need to rely on police, fire, and other officials for instructions. However, you can prepare in much the same way you would prepare for other crisis events.

General safety guidelines are as follows:

- Be aware of your surroundings.

- Move or leave if you feel uncomfortable or if something does not seem right.

♣ **It's A Fact!!**

Acts of terrorism include threats of terrorism; assassinations; kidnappings; hijackings; bomb scares and bombings; cyber attacks (computer-based); and the use of chemical, biological, nuclear, and radiological weapons.

Source: Federal Emergency Management Agency, April 2006.

- Take precautions when traveling. Be aware of conspicuous or unusual behavior. Do not accept packages from strangers. Do not leave luggage unattended. You should promptly report unusual behavior, suspicious or unattended packages, and strange devices to the police or security personnel.

- Learn where emergency exits are located in buildings you frequent. Plan how to get out in the event of an emergency.

- Be prepared to do without services you normally depend on—electricity, telephone, natural gas, gasoline pumps, cash registers, ATMs, and internet transactions.

- Work with building owners to ensure the following items are located on each floor of the building:

  - portable, battery-operated radio and extra batteries

  - several flashlights and extra batteries

  - first aid kit and manual

  - hard hats and dust masks

  - fluorescent tape to rope off dangerous areas

Explosions

Terrorists have frequently used explosive devices as one of their most common weapons. Terrorists do not have to look far to find out how to make explosive devices; the information is readily available in books and other information sources. The materials needed for an explosive device can be found in many places including variety, hardware, and auto supply stores. Explosive devices are highly portable using vehicles and humans as a means of transport. They are easily detonated from remote locations or by suicide bombers.

Conventional bombs have been used to damage and destroy financial, political, social, and religious institutions. Attacks have occurred in public places and on city streets with thousands of people around the world injured and killed.

Bomb Threat

If a person receives a telephoned bomb threat, he or she should do the following:

- Get as much information from the caller as possible. Try to ask the following questions:

    1. When is the bomb going to explode?
    2. Where is it right now?
    3. What does it look like?
    4. What kind of bomb is it?
    5. What will cause it to explode?
    6. Did you place the bomb?
    7. Why?
    8. What is your address?
    9. What is your name?

- Keep the caller on the line and record everything that is said.

- Notify the police and building management.

- If you do not have a container, then cover the envelope or package with anything available (e.g., clothing, paper, trash can, etc.) and do not remove the cover.

- Leave the room and close the door, or section off the area to prevent others from entering.

- Wash your hands with soap and water to prevent spreading any powder to your face.

- If you are at work, report the incident to your building security official or an available supervisor, who should notify police and other authorities without delay.

- List all people who were in the room or area when this suspicious letter or package was recognized. Give a copy of this list to both the local public health authorities and law enforcement officials for follow-up investigations and advice.

- If you are at home, report the incident to local police.

Biological Threats

Biological agents are organisms or toxins that can kill or incapacitate people, livestock, and crops. The three basic groups of biological agents that would likely be used as weapons are bacteria, viruses, and toxins. Most biological agents are difficult to grow and maintain. Many break down quickly when exposed to sunlight and other environmental factors, while others, such as anthrax spores, are very long-lived. Biological agents can be dispersed by spraying them into the air, by infecting animals that carry the disease to humans, and by contaminating food and water. Delivery methods include the following:

- **Aerosols:** Biological agents are dispersed into the air, forming a fine mist that may drift for miles. Inhaling the agent may cause disease in people or animals.

- **Animals:** Some diseases are spread by insects and animals such as fleas, mice, flies, mosquitoes, and livestock.

- **Food And Water Contamination:** Some pathogenic organisms and toxins may persist in food and water supplies. Most microbes can be killed, and toxins deactivated, by cooking food and boiling water. Boiling water for one minute kills most microbes, but some require longer. Follow official instructions.

- **Person-To-Person:** Spread of a few infectious agents is also possible. Humans have been the source of infection for smallpox, plague, and the Lassa viruses.

During A Biological Attack

In the event of a biological attack, public health officials may not immediately be able to provide information on what you should do. It will take time to determine what the illness is, how it should be treated, and who is in danger. Watch television, listen to the radio, or check the internet for official news and information including signs and symptoms of the disease, areas in danger, if medications or vaccinations are being distributed, and where you should seek medical attention if you become ill.

The first evidence of an attack may be when you notice symptoms of the disease caused by exposure to an agent. Be suspicious of any symptoms you notice, but do not assume that any illness is a result of the attack. Use common sense and practice good hygiene.

If you become aware of an unusual and suspicious substance nearby, do the following:

- Move away quickly.
- Wash with soap and water.
- Contact authorities.
- Listen to the media for official instructions.
- Seek medical attention if you become sick.

If you are exposed to a biological agent, do the following:

- Remove and bag your clothes and personal items. Follow official instructions for disposal of contaminated items.

- Wash yourself with soap and water and put on clean clothes.

- Seek medical assistance. You may be advised to stay away from others or even quarantined.

Using High Efficiency Particulate Air (HEPA) Filters

HEPA filters are useful in biological attacks. If you have a central heating and cooling system in your home with a HEPA filter, leave it on if it is running or turn the fan on if it is not running. Moving the air in the house through the filter will help remove the agents from the air. If you have a portable HEPA filter, take it with you to the internal room where you are seeking shelter and turn it on.

If you are in an apartment or office building that has a modern, central heating and cooling system, the system's filtration should provide a relatively safe level of protection from outside biological contaminants.

Chemical Threats

Chemical agents are poisonous vapors, aerosols, liquids, and solids that have toxic effects on people, animals, or plants. They can be released by bombs or sprayed from aircraft, boats, and vehicles. They can be used as a liquid to create a hazard to people and the environment. Some chemical agents may be odorless and tasteless. They can have an immediate effect (a few seconds to a few minutes) or a delayed effect (2 to 48 hours). While potentially lethal, chemical agents are difficult to deliver in lethal concentrations. Outdoors, the agents often dissipate rapidly. Chemical agents also are difficult to produce.

A chemical attack could come without warning. Signs of a chemical release include people having difficulty breathing; experiencing eye irritation; losing coordination; becoming nauseated; or having a burning sensation in the nose, throat, and lungs. Also, the presence of many dead insects or birds may indicate a chemical agent release.

> ✤ **It's A Fact!!**
> HEPA filters will not filter chemical agents.
>
> Source: Federal Emergency Management Agency, March 2006.

During A Chemical Attack

If you are instructed to remain in your home or office building, you should do the following:

• Close doors and windows and turn off all ventilation, including furnaces, air conditioners, vents, and fans.

• Seek shelter in an internal room and take your disaster supplies kit.

• Seal the room with duct tape and plastic sheeting.

• Listen to your radio for instructions from authorities.

If you are caught in or near a contaminated area, you should do the following:

• Move away immediately in a direction upwind of the source.

• Find shelter as quickly as possible.

Why do some teens want to hurt themselves?

Many people cut themselves because it gives them a sense of relief. Some people use cutting as a means to cope with any problem. Some teens say that when they hurt themselves, they are trying to stop feeling lonely, angry, or hopeless. Some teens that hurt themselves have low self-esteem, they may feel unloved by their family and friends, and they may have an eating disorder, an alcohol or drug problem, or may have been victims of abuse.

Teens who hurt themselves often keep their feelings "bottled up" inside and have a hard time letting their feelings show. Some teens that hurt themselves say that feeling the pain provides a sense of relief from intense feelings. Cutting can relieve the tension from bottled up sadness or anxiety. Others hurt themselves in order to "feel." Often people who hold back strong emotions can begin feeling numb, and cutting can be a way to cope with this because it causes them to feel something. Some teens also may hurt themselves because they want to fit in with others who do it.

Who are the people who hurt themselves?

People who hurt themselves come from all walks of life, no matter their age, gender, race, or ethnicity. About 1 in 100 people hurts himself or herself on purpose. More females hurt themselves than males. Teens usually hurt themselves by cutting with sharp objects.

What are the signs of self-injury?

These are some signs of self-injury:

• cuts or scars on the arms or legs

• hiding cuts or scars by wearing long sleeved shirts or pants, even in hot weather

• making poor excuses about how the injuries happened

Self-injury can be dangerous—cutting can lead to infections, scars, numbness, and even hospitalization and death.

☞ **Remember!!**

If you are hurting yourself, you need to get help. It is possible to overcome the urge to cut. There are other ways to find relief and cope with your emotions. Talk to your parents, your doctor, or an adult you trust, like a teacher or religious leader.

Source:
GirlsHealth.gov

People who share tools to cut themselves are at risk of getting, and spreading, diseases like human immunodeficiency virus (HIV) and hepatitis. Teens who continue to hurt themselves are less likely to learn how to cope with negative feelings.

Are you or a friend depressed, angry, or having a hard time?

If you are thinking about hurting yourself, you need to ask for help. Talk with an adult you trust, like a teacher, minister, or doctor. There is nothing wrong with asking for help—everyone needs help sometimes. You have a right to be strong, safe, and happy.

Do you have a friend who hurts herself or himself?

Try to get your friend to talk to a trusted adult. Your friend may need professional counseling and treatment. Help is available. Counselors can teach positive ways to cope with problems without turning to self-injury.

Have you been pressured to cut yourself by others who do it?

If so, think about how much you value that friendship or relationship. Do you really want a friend who wants you to hurt yourself, cause you pain, and put you in danger? Try to hang out with other friends who do not pressure you in this way.

How Is Self-Harm Treated?

Self-harm is a problem that many people are embarrassed or ashamed to discuss. Often, individuals try to hide their self-harm behaviors and are very reluctant to seek needed psychological or even medical treatment.

Psychological Treatments

Because self-harm is often associated with other psychological problems, it tends to be treated under the umbrella of a co-occurring disorder like a substance abuse problem or an eating disorder. Sometimes the underlying feelings that cause the self-harm are the same as those that cause the co-occurring disorder. For example, a person's underlying feelings of shame may cause them to abuse drugs and cut themselves. Often, the self-harm can be addressed in the context of therapy for an associated problem. For example, if people can learn healthy coping skills to help them deal with their urges to abuse substances, they may be able to apply these same skills to their urges to harm themselves.

There are also some treatments that specifically focus on stopping the self-harm. A good example of this is dialectical behavior therapy (DBT), a treatment that involves individual therapy and group skills training. DBT is a therapy approach that was originally developed for individuals with borderline personality disorder who engage in self-harm or "parasuicidal behaviors." Now the treatment is also being used for self-harming individuals with a wide variety of other psychological problems including eating disorders and substance dependence. The theory behind DBT is that individuals tend to engage in self-harm in an attempt to regulate or control their strong emotions. DBT teaches clients alternative ways of managing their emotions and tolerating distress. Research has shown that DBT is helpful in reducing self-harm.

Pharmacological Treatments

It is possible that psychopharmacological treatments would be helpful in reducing self-harm behaviors, but this has not yet been rigorously studied. As yet, there is no consensus regarding whether or not psychiatric medications should be used in relation to self-harm behaviors. This is a complicated issue to study because self-harm can occur in many different populations and co-occur with many different kinds of psychological problems. If you are wondering about the use of medications for the emotions related to your self-harm behaviors, it is recommended that you discuss this with your doctor or psychiatrist.

How To Find A Qualified Psychologist Or Psychiatrist

If you are trying to find a psychologist or psychiatrist, you should ask them if they are familiar with self-harm. Consider which issues are important to you and make sure you can talk to the potential therapist about them. Remember that you are the consumer and have the right to interview therapists until you find someone with whom you feel comfortable. You may want to ask trusted friends or medical professionals for referrals to psychologists or psychiatrists. Consider asking your potential provider questions such as the following:

• How do you treat self-harm?

• What do you think causes self-harm?

• Do you have experience in treating self-harm?

Chapter 31

Teen Suicide

Violence Against Self

Some people who have trouble dealing with their feelings don't react by lashing out at others. Instead, they direct violence toward themselves. The most final and devastating expression of this kind of violence is suicide.

Like people who are violent toward others, potential suicide victims often behave in recognizable ways before they try to end their lives. Suicide, like other forms of violence, is preventable. The two most important steps in prevention are recognizing warning signs and getting help.

Warning signs of potential self-violence include:

• previous suicide attempts

• significant alcohol or drug use

About This Chapter: This chapter begins with "Violence Against Self," from "Warning Signs of Youth Violence," http://www.apahelpcenter.org/dl/warning_signs-of_youth_violence.pdf, Copyright © 2002 by the American Psychological Association. Reprinted with permission. The official citation used in referencing this material is: American Psychological Association Practice Directorate, *Warning Signs of Youth Violence*, March 2002. The chapter continues with "Questions And Answers About Teen Suicide" from "Suicide," National Women's Health Information Center (GirlsHealth.gov), March 2006. It concludes with "Types of Suicide Prevention Programs," excerpted from "Youth Suicide Prevention Programs: A Resource Guide," Centers for Disease Control and Prevention (CDC), September 1992; http://wonder.cdc.gov, accessed January 2007. Despite the older date of this document, the descriptions of the different kinds of programs are still appropriate for readers seeking to understand this issue.

- threatening or communicating thoughts of suicide, death, dying, or the afterlife

- sudden increase in moodiness, withdrawal, or isolation

- major change in eating or sleeping habits

- feelings of hopelessness, guilt, or worthlessness

- poor control over behavior

- impulsive, aggressive behavior

- drop in quality of school performance or interest

- lack of interest in usual activity

- getting into trouble with authority figures

- perfectionism

- giving away important possessions

- hinting at not being around in the future or saying good-bye

These warning signs are especially noteworthy in the context of:

- a recent death or suicide of a friend or family member

- a recent break-up with a boyfriend or girlfriend, or conflict with parents

- news reports of other suicides by young people in the same school or community

Often, suicidal thinking comes from a wish to end deep psychological pain. Death seems like the only way out. But it isn't.

If a friend mentions suicide, take it seriously. Listen carefully, then seek help immediately. Never keep their talk of suicide a secret, even if they ask you to. Remember, you risk losing that person. Forever.

When you recognize the warning signs for suicidal behavior, do something about it. Tell a trusted adult what you have seen or heard. Get help from a licensed mental health professional as soon as possible. They can help work out the problems that seem so unsolvable but, in fact, are not.

Take a stand against violence.

Questions And Answers About Teen Suicide

Why do some teens think about suicide?

Thinking about suicide often goes along with stressful events and feeling sad. Some teens feel so overwhelmed and sad that they think they will never feel better. Some things that can cause these feelings include the following:

- death of a loved one

- seeing a lot of anger and violence at home

- having parents get divorced

- having a hard time in school, struggling with grades, or having problems with other teens

- depression or alcohol or drug problems

- anger or heartbreak over a relationship break-up

- feeling like you do not belong, either within the family or with friends

- feeling left out or alone

Sometimes teens may feel very sad for no one clear reason.

Every teen feels anxiety and confusion at some point, but it helps to get through tough times by turning to people you trust and love. If you do not think you have people like this in your life, talk to a school counselor, teacher, doctor, or another adult who can help you talk about your feelings. There are ways to help teens deal with these intense feelings and work on feeling better in the future.

How common is the problem of teen suicide?

Suicide is one of the leading causes of death for teens. Girls try to commit suicide more often than boys. The important thing for you to know is that it does not have to happen. It is also important to know that suicide is not a heroic act, even though sometimes media images can make it seem so. Often, a person who is thinking about attempting suicide is not able to see that suicide is never the answer to problems. Remember, there is always help, as well as support and love, out there for you or a friend.

How can you help a friend?

If you have a friend or friends who have talked about suicide, take it seriously. The first thing you should do is to tell an adult you trust right away. You may wonder if your friend(s) will be mad at you, but telling an adult is the right thing to do. This can be someone in your family, a coach, a school nurse, counselor, or a teacher. You can call 911 or the toll-free number of a suicide crisis line. You cannot help your friend(s) alone. They will need a good support system, including friends, family, teachers, and professional help. Suggest that they should talk with a trusted adult. Offer to listen and encourage them to talk about their feelings. Do not ignore their worries or tell them they will get better on their own. Listening shows that you take your friend(s) and their problems seriously and that you are there to help.

What about you?

If you feel suicidal, talk to an adult right away. Call 911 or 1-800-SUICIDE or check in your phone book for the number of a suicide crisis center. The centers offer experts who can help callers talk through their problems and develop a plan of action. These hotlines can also tell you where to go for more help in person.

☞ **Remember!!**

If someone is in danger of hurting himself or herself, do not leave the person alone. You may need to call 911.

Source: National Women's Health Information Center (GirlsHealth.gov)

Things may seem bad at times, but those times do not last forever. Your pain right now probably feels like it is too overwhelming to cope with—suicide may feel like the only form of relief, but remember that people do make it through suicidal thoughts. Ask for help. You can feel better. Do not use alcohol or drugs, because they cannot take your problems away. If you cannot find someone to talk with, write down your thoughts. Try to remember and write down the things you are grateful for. List the people who are your friends and family and care for you. Write about your hopes for the future. Read what you have written when you need to remind yourself that your life is important.

Remember!!

There is no reason that you or a friend has to continue hurting. There are ways to find help and hope.

Source: National Women's Health Information Center (GirlsHealth.gov)

What if someone you know attempts or dies by suicide?

If someone you know attempts or dies by suicide, it is important to remember that it is not your fault. You may feel many different emotions: anger, grief, guilt, or you may even feel numb. All of your feelings are okay; there is not a right or wrong way to feel. If you are having trouble dealing with your feelings, talk to a trusted adult. It is important that you feel strong ties with people at this time.

Types of Suicide Prevention Programs

There is a broad spectrum of youth suicide prevention programs ranging from general education about suicide to crisis center hotlines. The different prevention strategies are designed to prevent suicide in various ways. For example, gatekeeper training and screening programs are designed to identify people at risk of suicide and refer them to mental health services. Conversely, hotlines are intended to help people who are experiencing a crisis.

Eight different kinds of program activities representing different strategies for suicide prevention are described below. However, suicide prevention programs are typically quite comprehensive, incorporating several different strategies. For example, general suicide education programs in schools are almost always associated with gatekeeper training for school personnel. Similarly, in many communities, crisis center personnel conduct general suicide education programs. Many suicide prevention programs include several of these components in their activities, and many in the field believe that comprehensive programs offering multiple components facilitate the type of synergy and coordination that is more effective than any individual component.

School Gatekeeper Training: This type of program is directed at school staff (teachers, counselors, coaches, etc.) to help them identify students at risk of suicide and refer such students as appropriate. These programs also teach staff how to respond in cases of a tragic death or other crisis in the school.

Community Gatekeeper Training: This type of gatekeeper program provides training to community members, such as clergy, police, merchants, and recreation staff, as well as physicians, nurses, and other clinicians who see youthful patients. This training is designed to help these people identify youth at risk of suicide and refer them as appropriate.

General Suicide Education: These programs provide students with facts about suicide, alert them to suicide warning signs, and provide information about how to seek help for themselves or for others. These programs often incorporate a variety of self-esteem or social competency development activities.

Screening Programs: Screening involves the administration of an instrument to identify high-risk youth in order to provide more targeted assessment and treatment. Repeated administration of the screening instrument can also be used to measure changes in attitudes or behaviors over time to test the effectiveness of an employed prevention strategy and to obtain early warning signs of potential suicidal behavior.

Peer Support Programs: These programs, which can be conducted in either school or non-school settings, are designed to foster peer relationships, competency development, and social skills among youth at high risk of suicide or suicidal behavior.

Crisis Centers And Hotlines: Among other services, these programs primarily provide telephone counseling for suicidal people. Trained volunteers usually staff hotlines. Such programs may also offer a "drop-in" crisis center and referral to mental health services.

Means Restriction: This prevention strategy consists of activities designed to restrict access to handguns, drugs, and other common means of suicide.

Intervention After A Suicide: Strategies have been developed to cope with the crisis sometimes caused by one or more youth suicides in a community. They are designed in part to help prevent or contain suicide clusters and to help youth effectively cope with feelings of loss that come with the sudden death or suicide of a peer. Preventing further suicides is but one of several goals of interventions made with friends and relatives of a suicide victim—so-called "postvention" efforts.

Part Three

Recognizing And Treating The Consequences Of Abuse And Violence

Chapter 32

What To Do After A Sexual Assault

What Should I Do?

• Find a safe environment—anywhere away from the attacker. Ask a trusted friend to stay with you for moral support.

• Know that what happened was not your fault and that now you should do what is best for you.

• Report the attack to police by calling 911. A counselor on the National Sexual Assault Hotline at 1-800-656-HOPE can help you understand the process.

  • Preserve evidence of the attack—don't bathe or brush your teeth.

  • Write down all the details you can recall about the attack and the attacker.

  • Ask the hospital to conduct a rape kit exam to preserve forensic evidence.

About This Chapter: Information in this chapter begins with text from "What Should I Do," "Reporting Rape," "First Aid Tips," "Effects of Rape," "Post-Rape Medical Attention," "What is a SANE/SART," "Self-Care," and "Pregnancy from Rape." © 2006 Rape, Abuse and Incest National Network (www.rainn.org). Reprinted with permission. Information under the heading "Testing For STDs And HIV" is excerpted from "Sexual Assault," The United States Attorney's Office, Central District of California; retrieved June 2007.

- If you suspect you were drugged, ask that a urine sample be collected. The sample will need to be analyzed later on by a forensic lab.

- If you know that you will never report, still consider the following:

    - Get medical attention. Even with no physical injuries, it is important to determine the risks of STDs and pregnancy.

    - Call the National Sexual Assault Hotline, operated by Rape, Abuse and Incest National Network (RAINN), for free, confidential counseling, 24 hours a day: 1-800-656-HOPE.

- Recognize that healing from rape takes time. Give yourself the time you need.

- Know that it's never too late to call. Even if the attack happened years ago, the National Sexual Assault Hotline or the National Sexual Assault Online Hotline (http://www.rainn.org/ohl-bridge.php) can still help. Many victims do not realize they need help until months or years later.

Reporting Rape

Should I report my attack to the police?

We hope you will decide to report your attack to the police. While there's no way to change what happened to you, you can seek justice while helping to stop it from happening to someone else.

Reporting to the police is the key to preventing sexual assault. Every time we lock up a rapist, we're preventing him or her from committing another attack. It's the most effective tool that exists to prevent future rapes. In the end, though, whether or not to report is your decision to make.

Am I required to report to police?

No, you are not legally obligated to report. The decision is entirely yours, and everyone will understand if you decided not to pursue prosecution. (You should be aware that the district attorney's office retains the right to pursue prosecution whether or not you participate, though it is uncommon for them to proceed without the cooperation of the victim. There are also times when a third party, such as a doctor or teacher, is required to report a suspicion of sexual abuse.

Many victims say that reporting is the last thing they want to do right after being attacked. That's perfectly understandable—reporting can seem invasive, time consuming and difficult.

Still, there are many good reasons to report, and some victims say that reporting helped their recovery and helped them regain a feeling of control.

✔ Quick Tip
What To Do If You Have Been Sexually Assaulted

- Get away from the attacker to a safe place as fast as you can. Then call 911 or the police.

- Call a friend or family member you trust. You also can call a crisis center or a hotline to talk with a counselor. One hotline is the National Sexual Assault Hotline at 1-800-656-HOPE. Feelings of shame, guilt, fear, and shock are normal. It is important to get counseling from a trusted professional.

- Do not wash, comb, or clean any part of your body. Do not change clothes if possible, so the hospital staff can collect evidence. Do not touch or change anything at the scene of the assault.

- Go to your nearest hospital emergency room as soon as possible. You need to be examined, treated for any injuries, and screened for possible sexually transmitted diseases (STDs) or pregnancy. The doctor will collect evidence using a rape kit for fibers, hairs, saliva, semen, or clothing that the attacker may have left behind.

- You or the hospital staff can call the police from the emergency room to file a report.

- Ask the hospital staff about possible support groups you can attend right away.

Source: Excerpted from "Sexual Assault," The National Women's Health Information Center, U.S. Department of Health and Human Services, Office On Women's Health, January 2005.

How do I report the rape to police?

Call 911 (or ask a friend to call) to report your rape to police. Or, visit a hospital emergency room or your own doctor and ask them to call the police for you. If you visit the emergency room and tell the nurse you have been raped, the hospital will generally perform a sexual assault forensic examination. This involves collecting evidence of the attack, such as hairs, fluids and fibers, and preserving the evidence for forensic analysis. In most areas, the local rape crisis center can provide someone to accompany you, if you wish. Call 1-800-656-HOPE to contact the center in your area.

Is there a time limit on reporting to the police?

There's generally no legal barrier to reporting your attack even months afterwards. However, to maximize the chances of an arrest and successful prosecution, it's important that you report as soon as possible after the rape. If you aren't sure what to do, it's better to report now and decide later. That way, the evidence is preserved should you decide to pursue prosecution.

Some states have statutes of limitations that bar prosecutions after a certain number of years. View information on your state at http://www.ndaa-apri.org/apri/programs/vawa/statutes.html.

What if I need time to think about whether I want to pursue prosecution?

Understandably, many people aren't ready to make the decision about prosecution immediately after an attack. It's normal to want time to think about the decision and talk it over with friends and family.

If you think you might want to pursue prosecution, but haven't decided for sure, it is recommended that you make the police report right away, while the evidence is still present and your memory is still detailed. The district attorney will decide whether or not to pursue prosecution, however, it is unusual for cases to proceed without the cooperation of the victim. And if prosecution is pursued, the chance of success will be much higher if you reported, and had evidence collected, immediately after the attack.

There's one additional consideration: If you are planning to apply for compensation through your state's Victim Compensation Fund, you will generally first have to report your attack to police to be eligible. Contact your local rape crisis center at 1-800-656-HOPE to learn about the rules in your state.

Can I report to police even if I have no physical injuries?

Yes. In fact, most rapes do not result in physical injuries. So, the lack of such injuries should not deter you from reporting.

It's also important to get medical care and to be tested for sexually transmitted infections and pregnancy, even if you think you aren't injured. And keep in mind that rape can cause injuries, often internal, that aren't visible. Many hospitals have special equipment that can detect such hidden injuries.

The rapist got scared away before finishing the attack. Can I still report it?

Yes. Attempted rape is still a serious crime and should be reported.

I knew the person who raped me and invited him/her in. Can I still report it?

Yes. About two-thirds of victims know their attacker. And the fact that you were voluntarily together, or even invited him/her home with you, does not change anything. Rape is a serious crime, no matter what the circumstances.

Do I have to go through the police interview alone?

In most areas, a trained volunteer from your local rape crisis center can accompany you to the police interview. The volunteer can also answer your questions about the process and explain how it will work. To reach your local crisis center, call 1-800-656-HOPE.

What's the reporting process?

In most cases, the police will come to you and take a statement about what occurred. It helps to write down every detail you can remember, as soon as possible, so you can communicate the details to the police.

I'm afraid of getting in trouble.

Sometimes victims, particularly youth, are afraid of getting in trouble for doing something they weren't supposed to be doing when the assault took place, such as drinking or sneaking out. While there's a possibility that you can get in trouble, most authorities (and parents) will be understanding, particularly about minor infractions.

✎ What's It Mean?

First Responder: A professional who initially responds to a disclosure of a sexual assault (there is often more than one first responder). These professionals typically must follow agency-specific policies for responding to victims. Those who traditionally have been responsible for immediate response to adult and adolescent sexual assaults include victim advocates, 911 dispatchers, law enforcement representatives, and health care providers.

Forensic Scientist: Responsible for analyzing evidence in sexual assault cases. This evidence typically includes DNA and other biological evidence, toxicology samples, latent prints, and trace evidence.

Law Enforcement Representative: Different types of law enforcement agencies exist at the local, state, territory, tribal, and federal levels. Any of these agencies could potentially be involved in responding to sexual assault cases. Also, in areas without a local law enforcement agency, public safety officials may assist in immediate response to sexual assault victims. Some agencies may have staff with specialized education and experience in sexual assault investigations.

Sexual Assault: The sexual contact of one person with another without appropriate legal consent. This definition includes, but is not limited to, a wide range of behavior classified by state, territory, federal, and tribal law as rape, sexual assault, sexual misconduct, and sexual battery.

Sexual Assault Medical Forensic Examination: An examination of a sexual assault patient by a health care provider, ideally one who has specialized education and clinical experience in the collection of forensic evidence and treatment of these patients. The forensic component includes gathering information from

What if I decide not to report?

Reporting is a very personal decision, and you should make the decision that's right for you. While we encourage you to report, if you decide not to, for whatever reason, that's perfectly understandable and there's no reason to feel bad about your decision.

the patient for the medical forensic history, an examination, documentation of biological and physical findings, collection of evidence from the patient, and follow-up as needed to document additional evidence. The medical component includes coordinating treatment of injuries, providing care for STIs, assessing pregnancy risk, and discussing treatment options, including reproductive health services, and providing instructions and referrals for follow-up medical care.

Sexual Assault Response Team (SART): A multidisciplinary team that provides specialized immediate response to victims of recent sexual assault. The team typically includes health care personnel, law enforcement representatives, victim advocates, prosecutors (usually available on-call to consult with first responders, although some may be more actively involved at this stage), and forensic lab personnel (typically available to consult with examiners, law enforcement, or prosecutors, but not actively involved at this stage).

Victim Service Provider/Advocate: May offer victims and their significant others a range of services during the exam process. These services may include support, crisis intervention, information and referrals, and advocacy to ensure that victims' interests are represented, their wishes respected, and their rights upheld. In addition, advocates and other victim service providers may provide follow-up services, such as support groups, counseling, accompaniment to related appointments, and legal advocacy to help meet the needs of victims, their families, and friends.

Source: Excerpted from *A National Protocol for Sexual Assault Medical Forensic Examinations: Adults/Adolescents*, Publication NCJ 206554, Office on Violence Against Women, U.S. Department of Justice, September 2004.

First Aid Tips

The following first aid tips may be helpful if you or someone you know has recently been assaulted. While these tips can help to avoid infections from minor cuts and bruises, going to the hospital for a more complete check up for further injuries is very important.

👉 **Remember!!**

A victim of sexual assault should wait to bathe or change their clothes until he or she can go to a hospital for a complete examination to preserve evidence of the crime. Furthermore, if the victim suspects that he or she has been drugged, try to preserve his or her first urine sample.

Source: Excerpted from "First Aid Tips." © 2006 Rape, Abuse and Incest National Network (www.rainn.org). Reprinted with permission.

Treating A Black Eye

• Apply a cold pack or ice-filled cloth to reduce swelling. Continue for up to two days after the injury.

• Check for blood in any part of the eye.

• Go to the emergency room if there is any bleeding in the eye, bleeding from the nose, vision problems, or severe pain.

Treating Bruises

• You don't need a bandage, but you can enhance healing by elevating the injured area and applying ice or a cold pack, 30 to 60 minutes at a time for up to two days.

• Take acetaminophen (Tylenol).

• Contact a doctor if you're experiencing abnormal bleeding, such as from the nose, gums, eyes, urine, or excrement.

Treating Cuts And Scrapes

• Stop the bleeding. Usually, cuts and scrapes will stop bleeding on their own. If not, apply pressure with a clean cloth. Hold pressure for 20 to 30 minutes. Do not keep checking to see if the bleeding has stopped because this may damage the fresh clot while it's forming.

- Clean the wound. Rinse out with plain water; soap can irritate wounds. Use tweezers to remove any remaining dirt or debris or contact a doctor if you're unable to remove it yourself. Clean the wound thoroughly to avoid tetanus. There's no need for hydrogen peroxide or iodine, but if you use them, don't apply directly to the wound because they irritate living cells.

- Apply antibiotic. Apply a thin layer of antibiotic cream or ointment like Neosporin or Polysporin to help keep the surface moist. This discourages infection and increases the effectiveness of healing, though it does not speed up the healing process.

- Cover the wound. Bandages help keep the wound clean and prevent infection.

- Watch for signs of infection. See your doctor if the wound is not healing or if you notice redness, drainage, warmth, or swelling. Also, doctors recommend that you get a tetanus shot every ten years. If your wound is deep or dirty, and your last shot was more than five years ago, a booster may be needed. Get the booster within 48 hours of injury.

Post-Rape Medical Attention

While the biggest scars from your attack are likely to be emotional, there may be physical consequences as well. So, it is important to get prompt medical attention.

- Make sure that all your cuts, bruises, broken bones, etc. are taken care of.

- Even if there are no physical injuries, it is important to determine the risks of pregnancy and sexually transmitted infections (STIs), including human immunodeficiency virus (HIV). This may require follow-up testing in addition to your initial treatment.

- The hospital is the best place to collect forensic evidence of your attack. Many hospitals have nurses called SANEs (sexual assault nurse examiners) or SAFEs (sexual assault forensic examiners), who are specially trained to collect evidence from rape victims. This evidence is crucial to the successful prosecution of your case.

- Ask your local hospital if they have a SANE nurse available, or call your local crisis center at 1-800-656-HOPE to find out which hospitals have SANEs in your area.

- Even if your hospital does not have a SANE nurse, make sure to ask the doctor or nurse to perform a "rape kit," which means they will collect fibers, hair, and other forensic evidence to preserve it for trial.

- Even if you are unsure if you want to pursue prosecution, it is important to collect this evidence before it is destroyed. Evidence collection does not commit you to prosecute—you can always change your mind later. But if you do not have the evidence collected right after the attack, it will most likely be lost. That will make it more difficult, or even impossible, to pursue prosecution later.

What Is A Rape Kit?

A rape kit is a standard kit with little boxes, microscope slides, and plastic bags for collecting and storing evidence. This process preserves evidence so that it may later be tested for DNA and used in court. The process involves collecting evidence left on your body and your clothing, including hair and fibers. It's a good idea to bring a change of clothing with you to the hospital, so you can put on fresh clothes after the evidence kit is completed.

✔ Quick Tip

If you suspect that you have been drugged, ask for a urine sample to be collected. The hospital will send the sample to a forensic lab to be analyzed. (This is not a part of a standard rape kit, so make sure to request it if appropriate.)

Source: From "Post-Rape Medical Attention," © 2006 Rape, Abuse and Incest National Network (www.rainn.org).

What Is A SANE/SART?

If you have been recently sexually assaulted and decide to complete a rape kit, you may hear the terms SANE or SART. These are important resources to know about if following a sexual assault you are seeking any sort of medical attention or if you are considering reporting the crime. It is important to note that these services may or may not be available in your local area. To find out, please contact your local crisis center.

Who is a SANE?

A Sexual Assault Nurse Examiner (SANE) is a Registered Nurse who has received special training in providing comprehensive care to sexual assault victims. In addition, a SANE can conduct a forensic exam and may provide expert testimony at trial.

What is a SART?

The Sexual Assault Response Team (SART) is a community-based team that coordinates the response to victims of sexual assault. The team may be comprised of SANEs, hospital personnel, sexual assault victim advocates, law enforcement, prosecutors, judges, and any other professionals with a specific interest in assisting victims of sexual assault.

Effects Of Rape

It is helpful to receive counseling and treatment after experiencing a sexual assault to start the healing process and avoid dealing with the trauma in unhealthy ways. According to The World Report on Violence and Health (WHO, 2002), in the absence of trauma counseling, negative psychological effects have been known to persist for at least a year following a rape.

Rape-Related Post Traumatic Stress Disorder

Many rape victims experience what is referred to as rape-related post traumatic stress disorder (also called rape trauma syndrome). The four major symptoms of this are the following:

1. **Re-Experiencing The Trauma:** Rape victims may experience recurrent nightmares about the rape, flashbacks, or may have an inability to stop remembering the rape.

2. **Social Withdrawal:** This symptom has been called "psychic numbing" and involves not experiencing feelings of any kind.

3. **Avoidance Behaviors And Actions:** Victims may desire to avoid any feelings or thoughts that might recall to mind events about the rape.

- Seeking out situations in which you feel unsafe

- Taking actions that undermine your self-worth

- Using food and unhealthy eating as a way to control your body and emotional state

- Inflicting harm on your body

- Blaming yourself for what happened

Pregnancy From Rape

If you were recently raped, you may have concerns about becoming pregnant from the attack. If the assault happened a long time ago, you may have concerns about a pregnancy that resulted from the assault.

If You Were Recently Assaulted

- The decision of what to do is yours to make.

- If you need additional information in order to make a decision, consider the following:

  - Talking to your doctor

  - Talking to your spouse or partner

  - Talking to your spiritual leader

  - Looking at resources on the American Pregnancy Association website (http://www.americanpregnancy.org) or calling their helpline at 1-800-672-2296

If You Were Assaulted In The Past

If you were assaulted in the past and there was a resulting pregnancy, you may have some residual feelings about the pregnancy. It is important to understand that any of these (and other) feelings are normal, and that if you want to discuss them further, you can call the National Sexual Assault Hotline at 1-800-656-HOPE or contact the National Sexual Assault Online Hotline (http://www.rainn.org/ohl-bridge.php).

Feelings You Might Have

If You Chose To Have An Abortion

- You may regret the decision.

- You may wonder what would have happened.

- You may think it was the right decision for you to make at the time, but still sad.

- You may be at peace with the decision.

If You Were Forced To Have An Abortion

- You may be sad or angry about that decision.

- You may believe it was the right decision at the time, but still be sad or angry.

- You may be at peace with the decision.

If You Put The Baby Up For Adoption

- You may wonder what happened to the child.

- You may feel guilty about the decision.

- You may think it was the right decision at the time, but still be sad or wonder what happened to the child.

- You may be at peace with the decision.

If You Kept The Baby

- You may have fears that the child will be like your rapist.

- You may have ambiguous feelings about the baby/child.

- You may be concerned about how to tell the child.

- You may be at peace with the decision.

Testing For STDs And HIV

If you did not get immediate medical attention after the sexual assault, get a full check up for STDs, including HIV, right away. A rape examination usually includes STD tests. If STD and HIV testing are not available, you should go to another clinic for a test as soon as possible.

Most medical clinics, hospitals, and private physicians will test for STDs and HIV. Some clinics and public hospitals will do the testing free of charge. If the case is being investigated or prosecuted by a federal government agency, you are entitled to testing at no cost to you. Certain requirements apply. Check with the Victim Witness Assistance Program with the investigative agency investigating your case, or the Victim Witness Assistance Program at the U.S. Attorney's Office, for details and procedures. Many STDs take several days to several months to show up. If an STD is diagnosed at an exam done right after the assault, you probably had the STD before the assault. The infection could be from past sexual contact or drug use. Talk to your health care provider about taking medicine and telling partners. If your first tests are negative, you may be able to rule out the possibility that you had an STD before the assault.

Even if your tests are negative, get tested again in three to six months. You cannot be sure if you have HIV or another STD unless you get tested at least three months after the assault. It can take up to six months after infection for antibodies to show up on a test. Victim Assistance staff can assist you in obtaining this second test at no cost to you. Your health and peace of mind are worth it.

♣ It's A Fact!!
Testing And Confidentiality

It is important to be tested in a facility that offers counseling and protects your confidentiality. STD and HIV tests usually are free in public health clinics.

You have the right to have up to two confidential and anonymous tests following a sexual assault that poses a risk of transmission of HIV virus or an STD. Test results are not given over the phone or sent in the mail. The nurse who drew your blood will give you the test results on your second visit and explain them to you in private.

Source: The United States Attorney's Office, Central District of California.

While waiting for the test results, it is normal to feel anxious and worried. Your counselor or doctor may be able to help. During this time, you need to protect your health and your loved ones from infection.

Counseling And Information

Most sexual assault crisis centers have hotlines operated by trained counselors who understand sexual assault and will talk to you confidentially. Most medical centers also provide counseling or a Victim Witness Advocate from the investigative agency or U.S. Attorney's Office will help you make arrangements for counseling.

HIV Testing And The Perpetrator Of Sexual Assault

A judge can order a person charged with a sexual assault to be tested for HIV if the victim requests this through the Assistant U.S. Attorney. You will be given the results; however, you are allowed to share this information only with your doctor, counselor, family members, and any sexual partners you may have had after the assault.

Regardless of the perpetrator's test, you still need to have your own HIV test. Even if the perpetrator has HIV, you may not have been infected during the sexual assault. If the perpetrator's HIV test is negative, the perpetrator could still have HIV. Recent infections (within 3–6 months) may not show up on his test. People with HIV can infect others at any time, even before their own blood shows signs of HIV.

What You Need To Know About HIV And Other Sexually Transmitted Diseases

- There are many common sexually transmitted diseases (STDs), including gonorrhea, syphilis, chlamydia, genital warts, herpes, and HIV—the acquired immune deficiency syndrome (AIDS) virus.

- Proper testing is the only way to know if you are infected.

- STDs, including HIV, usually are passed through vaginal, oral, or anal intercourse. However, some STDs can be passed from skin-to-skin contact in the genital area.

- An infected woman can pass HIV to her baby through breast milk.

- Many STDs can be cured easily, especially if they are found early.

- HIV is fairly hard to get from a single sexual act.

- There are only a few cases of HIV infection from sexual assault.

- You are more likely to get other STDs from a single contact with an infected person.

- Signs of STDs may not show up right away. Some people never notice any signs of infection. This is especially true for women.

Chapter 33

Long-Term Consequences Of Child Abuse And Neglect

An estimated 872,000 children were victims of child abuse or neglect in 2004 (U.S. Department of Health and Human Services, 2006). While physical injuries may or may not be immediately visible, abuse and neglect can have consequences for children, families, and society that last lifetimes, if not generations.

The impact of child abuse and neglect is often discussed in terms of physical, psychological, behavioral, and societal consequences. In reality, however, it is impossible to separate them completely. Physical consequences, such as damage to a child's growing brain, can have psychological implications, such as cognitive delays or emotional difficulties. Psychological problems often manifest as high-risk behaviors. Depression and anxiety, for example, may make a person more likely to smoke, abuse alcohol or illicit drugs, or overeat. High-risk behaviors, in turn, can lead to long-term physical health problems such as sexually transmitted diseases, cancer, and obesity.

This chapter provides an overview of some of the most common physical, psychological, behavioral, and societal consequences of child abuse and neglect, while acknowledging that much crossover among categories exists.

About This Chapter: Information in this chapter is from "Long-term Consequences of Child Abuse and Neglect," July 2006, Child Welfare Information Gateway (www.childwelfare.gov), Children's Bureau, Administration for Children, Youth and Families, U.S. Department of Health and Human Services, July 2006.

Factors Affecting The Consequences Of Child Abuse

Not all abused and neglected children will experience long-term consequences. Outcomes of individual cases vary widely and are affected by a combination of factors including the following:

• the child's age and developmental status when the abuse or neglect occurred

• the type of abuse (physical abuse, neglect, sexual abuse, etc.)

• frequency, duration, and severity of abuse

• the relationship between the victim and his or her abuser

Researchers also have begun to explore why, given similar conditions, some children experience long-term consequences of abuse and neglect while others emerge relatively unscathed. The ability to cope, and even thrive, following a negative experience is sometimes referred to as "resilience." A number of protective factors may contribute to an abused or neglected child's resilience. These include individual characteristics such as optimism, self-esteem, intelligence, creativity, humor, and independence. Protective factors can also include the family or social environment such as a child's access to social support; in particular, a caring adult in the child's life can be an important protective factor. Community well-being, including neighborhood stability and access to health care, is also a protective factor.

Physical Health Consequences

The immediate physical effects of abuse or neglect can be relatively minor (bruises or cuts) or severe (broken bones, hemorrhage, or even death). In some cases the physical effects are temporary; however, the pain and suffering they cause a child should not be discounted. Meanwhile, the long-term impact of child abuse and neglect on physical health is just beginning to be explored. The following are some outcomes researchers have identified:

• **Shaken Baby Syndrome:** The immediate effects of shaking a baby, which is a common form of child abuse in infants, can include vomiting, concussion, respiratory distress, seizures, and death. Long-term consequences can include blindness, learning disabilities, mental retardation, cerebral palsy, or paralysis.

- **Impaired Brain Development:** Child abuse and neglect have been shown, in some cases, to cause important regions of the brain to fail to form properly, resulting in impaired physical, mental, and emotional development. In other cases, the stress of chronic abuse causes a "hyper arousal" response by certain areas of the brain, which may result in hyperactivity, sleep disturbances, and anxiety, as well as increased vulnerability to post-traumatic stress disorder, attention deficit/hyperactivity disorder, conduct disorder, and learning and memory difficulties.

- **Poor Physical Health:** A study of 700 children who had been in foster care for one year found that more than one-quarter of the children had some kind of recurring physical or mental health problem. A study of 9,500 Health Maintenance Organization participants showed a relationship between various forms of household dysfunction (including childhood abuse) and long-term health problems such as sexually transmitted diseases, heart disease, cancer, chronic lung disease, skeletal fractures, and liver disease.

Psychological Consequences

Researchers have identified links between child abuse and neglect and the following:

- **Poor Mental And Emotional Health:** In one long-term study, as many as 80 percent of young adults who had been abused met the diagnostic criteria for at least one psychiatric disorder at age 21. These young adults exhibited many problems including depression, anxiety, eating disorders, and suicide attempts. Other psychological and emotional conditions associated with abuse and neglect include panic disorder, dissociative disorders, attention deficit/hyperactivity disorder, posttraumatic stress disorder, and reactive attachment disorder.

✤ **It's A Fact!!**
The immediate emotional effects of abuse and neglect—isolation, fear, and an inability to trust—can translate into lifelong consequences including low self-esteem, depression, and relationship difficulties.

- **Cognitive Difficulties:** The National Survey of Child and Adolescent Well-Being found that children placed in out-of-home care due to abuse or neglect tended to score lower than the general population on measures of cognitive capacity, language development, and academic achievement.

- **Social Difficulties:** Children who are abused and neglected by caretakers often do not form secure attachments to them. These early attachment difficulties can lead to later difficulties in relationships with other adults as well as with peers.

Behavioral Consequences

Not all victims of child abuse and neglect will experience behavioral consequences; however, child abuse and neglect appear to make the following more likely:

- **Difficulties During Adolescence:** Studies have found abused and neglected children to be at least 25 percent more likely to experience problems such as delinquency, teen pregnancy, low academic achievement, drug use, and mental health problems.

- **Juvenile Delinquency And Adult Criminality:** A National Institute of Justice study indicated being abused or neglected as a child increased the likelihood of arrest as a juvenile by 59 percent. Abuse and neglect increased the likelihood of adult criminal behavior by 28 percent and violent crime by 30 percent.

- **Alcohol And Other Drug Abuse:** Research consistently reflects an increased likelihood that abused and neglected children will smoke cigarettes, abuse alcohol, or take illicit drugs. According to a report from the National Institute on Drug Abuse, as many as two-thirds of people in drug treatment programs reported being abused as children.

- **Abusive Behavior:** Abusive parents often have experienced abuse during their own childhoods. It is estimated approximately one-third of abused and neglected children will eventually victimize their own children.

Societal Consequences

While child abuse and neglect almost always occur within the family, the impact does not end there. Society as a whole pays a price for child abuse and neglect in terms of both direct and indirect costs as shown in the following:

- **Direct Costs:** Direct costs include those associated with maintaining a child welfare system to investigate allegations of child abuse and neglect, as well as expenditures by the judicial, law enforcement, health, and mental health systems to respond to and treat abused children and their families. A 2001 report by Prevent Child Abuse America estimates these costs at $24 billion per year.

- **Indirect Costs:** Indirect costs represent the long-term economic consequences of child abuse and neglect. These include juvenile and adult criminal activity, mental illness, substance abuse, and domestic violence. They can also include loss of productivity due to unemployment and underemployment, the cost of special education services, and increased use of the health care system. Prevent Child Abuse America recently estimated these costs at more than $69 billion per year (2001).

Chapter 34

Seeking Mental Health Services

Eric went to therapy two years ago when his parents were getting divorced. Although he no longer goes, he feels the two months he spent in therapy helped him get through the tough times as his parents worked out their differences. Melody began seeing her therapist a year ago when she was being bullied at school. She still goes every two weeks because she feels her therapy is really helping to build her self-esteem. And Britt just joined a therapy group for eating disorders led by her school's psychologist.

When our parents were in school, very few kids went to therapy. Now it's much more accepted, and lots of teens wonder if therapy could help them, too.

What are some reasons that teens go to therapists?

Sometimes people who are trying as hard as they can to get through a rough time, such as family troubles or problems in school, find that they just can't cope by themselves. They may be feeling sad, angry, or overwhelmed by what's been happening—and need help sorting out their feelings, finding solutions to their problems, or just feeling better. That's when therapy can help.

About This Chapter: Information in this chapter is from "Going to a Therapist." This information was provided by TeensHealth, one of the largest resources online for medically reviewed health information written for teens, kids, and parents. For more articles like this one, visit www.TeensHealth.org, or www.KidsHealth.org. © 2004 The Nemours Foundation.

Here are just a few examples of situations in which therapy can help someone work through problems:

- Working with a therapist can help someone overcome depression, anxiety, painful shyness, or an eating disorder.

- Working with a therapist can help a person who cuts or self-injures.

- Psychotherapy can help someone manage an attention problem or a learning problem.

- People in therapy can learn to deal with the emotional side of a weight problem or a chronic illness.

- Psychotherapy can help someone whose parents are going through a separation or divorce to sort through the many feelings these changes bring.

- Therapy can help someone who has experienced a trauma, a difficult loss, or the death of someone close.

- Working with a therapist can help a family troubled by too much fighting or anger, or one struggling with alcoholism or other addiction problem.

- Therapy can help teens sort out common problems such as peer pressure, and it can help build self-confidence and development of friendship skills.

- Therapy can offer someone support through a difficult time.

- Therapy can help people manage their anger or to learn to get along better with others.

Making the decision to seek help for a problem can be hard at first. It may be your idea to go to therapy because of a problem you're having that you want to get help with. Other times, parents or teachers might bring up the idea first because they have noticed that someone they care about is dealing with a difficult situation, is losing weight, or seems unusually sad, worried, angry, or upset. Some people in this situation might welcome the idea or even feel relieved. Others might feel criticized or might not be sure about getting help at first.

Sometimes people are told by teachers or parents that they have to go see a therapist—because they have been behaving in ways that are unacceptable, self-destructive, dangerous, or worrisome. When therapy is someone else's idea at first, a person may feel like resisting the whole idea. But learning a bit more about what therapy involves and what to expect can help make it seem like a good thing after all.

What is therapy?

Therapy is the treatment of a disorder or illness. Therapy isn't just for mental health, of course—you've probably heard people discussing other types of medical therapy, such as physical therapy or chemotherapy. But the word "therapy" is most often used to mean psychotherapy (sometimes called "talk therapy")—the psychological treatment of emotional and behavioral problems.

Psychotherapy is a process that's a lot like learning. Through therapy, people learn about themselves. They discover ways to overcome troubling feelings or behaviors, develop inner strengths or skills, or make changes in themselves or their situations.

A psychotherapist (therapist for short) is a person who has been professionally trained to help people with their emotional and behavioral problems. Psychiatrists, psychologists, social workers, counselors, and school psychologists are the titles of some of the licensed professionals who work as therapists. The letters following a therapist's name (for example, MD, PhD, EdD, MA, LCSW, LPC) refer to the particular education and degree that therapist has received.

Some therapists specialize in working with a certain age group or on a particular type of problem. Other therapists treat a mix of ages and issues. Some therapists work in hospitals, clinics, or counseling centers. Others work in schools or in psychotherapy offices.

What do therapists do?

Most therapy is a combination of talking and listening, building trust, and receiving support and guidance.

Through talking, listening, and observing, a therapist is able to evaluate the problem situation that needs attention and care. In doing so, the therapist can help a person figure out what's been making him or her so unhappy and how to get things going on a better track again.

It might take a few meetings with a therapist before a person decides to talk openly. Trust is the most important ingredient in therapy—after all, therapy involves being open and honest with someone and talking about sensitive topics like feelings, ideas, relationships, problems, disappointments,

---

♣ It's A Fact!!
Adolescent Access To Confidential Health Services

Physicians strongly support adolescents' access to confidential health services. An American Medical Association (AMA) survey found that physicians were even more likely than the general public to favor confidentiality for adolescent patients. For example, pediatricians described confidentiality as essential to obtaining necessary and factual information from their adolescent patients. A regional survey of pediatricians showed strong support of confidential health services for adolescents. The results were as follows:

- Seventy-five percent favored confidential treatment for adolescents.

- Forty-five percent unconditionally favored confidential treatment of adolescents, even when it meant withholding information from parents.

The issues surrounding confidentiality for minors are not covered comprehensively in the myriad state and federal statutes and regulations. Many states, however, have laws mandating that parents be notified of specific treatments or diagnoses given to minors.

Parental notification laws contain a variety of standards for disclosure of information by health care providers. In some cases, the provider has discretion whether to notify the parent of a minor's treatment. A few states allow disclosure of medical information to parents or guardians without the consent—and over the specific objection of—the minor patient. Other states provide guidance to health care providers for when a minor's medical information may be disclosed.

and hopes. A therapist is trained to be patient with people who need to take their own time talking about themselves and their situation.

Most of the time, a person meets with a therapist one on one, which is known as individual therapy. Sometimes, though, a therapist might work with a family (called family therapy) or a group of people who all are dealing with similar issues (called group therapy or a support group). Family therapy gives family members a chance to talk together with a therapist about problems that involve them all. Group therapy and support groups help people

These laws elevate the interests of the parent or guardian above those of the adolescent patient. By making a minor's health information available to the parent, the laws may well discourage teens from seeking needed care. An adolescent with a sexually transmitted disease, for instance, may forego treatment rather than risk a parent's embarrassment, disapproval, or violence. Many teens live in dysfunctional family environments, and parental involvement laws cannot transform these families into stable homes. As a Justice of the California Supreme Court has noted, "Not every pregnant adolescent has parents out of the comforting and idyllic world of Norman Rockwell."

Recognizing that reality, many states have statutes to protect teen confidentiality for specific services—particularly reproductive and sexual health, mental health, and drug and alcohol treatment. Protecting adolescent confidentiality for these services encourages teens to seek treatment for conditions that they may want to keep private from parents. Nothing in these statutes prevents teens from involving parents in health care decision-making, which most adolescents do.

Similar protections are guaranteed in other states for minors seeking treatment or testing for sexually transmitted diseases or for mental and psychological problems. In situations where parental notification might deter adolescents from seeking these essential health services, states have determined that protecting the minor's confidentiality is more important than promoting parental control and family autonomy.

Source: "Adolescent Access to Confidential Health Services," © 1997 Advocates for Youth. All rights reserved. Reprinted with permission. Despite the older date of this document, the information presented is still appropriate for readers seeking to understand adolescent access to confidential health services.

give and receive support and learn from each other and their therapist by discussing the issues they have in common.

What happens during therapy?

If you see a therapist, he or she will talk with you about your feelings, thoughts, relationships, and important values. At the beginning, therapy sessions are focused on discussing what you'd like to work on and setting goals. Some of the goals people in therapy may set include things like the following:

> ✔ **Quick Tip**
> Sticking to the schedule you agree on with your therapist and going to your appointments will ensure you have enough time with your therapist to work out your concerns. If your therapist suggests a schedule that you don't think you'll be able to keep, be up front about it so you can work out an alternative.
>
> Source: © 2004 The Nemours Foundation.

- improving self-esteem and gaining confidence

- feeling less depressed or less anxious

- doing better with friends or schoolwork

- learning to relate without arguing and managing anger

- making healthier choices (for example, about relationships or eating) and ending self-defeating behaviors

During the first visit, your therapist will probably ask you to talk a bit about yourself. This helps the therapist understand you better. The therapist will ask about the problems, concerns, and symptoms that you're having.

After one or two sessions, the therapist will probably explain his or her understanding of your situation, how therapy could help, and what the process will involve. Together, you and your therapist will decide on the goals for therapy and how frequently to meet. This may be once a week, every other week, or once a month.

Once the therapist has a full understanding of your situation, he or she might teach you new skills or help you to think about a situation in a new way. For example, therapists can help people develop better relationship skills or coping skills, including ways to build confidence, express feelings, or manage anger.

How private is it?

Therapists respect the privacy of their clients, and they keep things they're told confidential. A therapist won't tell anyone else—including parents—about what a person discusses in his or her sessions unless that person gives permission. The only exception is if therapists believe their clients may harm themselves or others. If the issue of privacy and confidentiality worries you, be sure to ask your therapist about it during your first meeting. It's important to feel comfortable with your therapist so you can talk openly about your situation.

Does it mean I'm crazy (or a freak)?

No. In fact, many people in your class have probably seen a therapist at some point—just like students often see tutors or coaches for extra help with schoolwork or sports. Getting help with an emotional problem is the same as getting help with a medical problem like asthma or diabetes.

There's nothing wrong with asking for help when you're faced with problems you can't solve alone. In fact, it's just the opposite. It takes a lot of courage and maturity to look for solutions to problems instead of ignoring or hiding them and allowing them to become worse. If you think that therapy could help you with a problem, ask an adult you trust—like a parent, school counselor, or doctor—to help you find a therapist.

A few adults still resist the idea of therapy because they don't fully understand it or have outdated ideas about it. A couple of generations ago, people didn't know as much about the mind or the mind-body connection as they do today, and people were left to struggle with their problems on their own. It used to be that therapy was only available to those with the most serious mental health problems, but that's no longer the case.

Therapy is helpful to people of all ages and with problems that range from mild to much more serious. Some people still hold onto old beliefs about therapy, such as thinking that teens "will grow out of" their problems. If the adults in your life don't seem open to talking about therapy, mention your concerns to a school counselor, coach, or doctor.

You don't have to hide the fact that you're going to a therapist, but you also don't have to tell anyone if you'd prefer not to. Some people find that

People experience depression differently, and they may show different symptoms. Sometimes it can be hard to tell the difference between typical teen behavior and this mental health problem. How do you know when something really is wrong? If you are showing four or more of these symptoms for longer than two weeks, you may be suffering from depression.

If you think you might be suffering from depression, look for these signs:

- a major change in eating and/or sleeping patterns—either an increase or a decrease

- frequent complaints of physical illness such as headaches and stomachaches

- low energy

- poor concentration

- thoughts or expressions of suicide or self-destructive behavior

- difficulty making decisions

- frequent sadness, tearfulness, or crying

- empty or hopeless feelings

- feelings of inadequacy, unworthiness, guilt

- extreme sensitivity to rejection or failure

- increased irritability, anger, or hostility

- decreased interest in activities or inability to enjoy former favorite activities

- persistent boredom

- withdrawal from other people

- lack of communication with others

- difficulty with relationships

- frequent absences from school or poor performance in school

- talk of or efforts to run away from home

Some of the risk factors include a family history of depression; extreme stress or sadness; use of alcohol or drugs; and difficulties in dealing with sexual orientation, a chronic illness, difficult relationships, financial problems, or any major unwelcome change.

Some people face depression once in a lifetime; others have it several times. Symptoms can be so severe that a person is unable to function as usual.

A less common type of depression, bipolar illness, has cycles of severe "lows" (symptoms of depression) and inappropriate "highs" (mania). Symptoms of mania include decreased need for sleep; increased energy and activity; increased talking and moving; poor judgment; inappropriate social behavior; disconnected and racing thoughts; inability to make decisions; flamboyant ideas; and inappropriate elation.

Diagnosis involves a thorough checkup that includes a complete physical exam and medical workup as well as a complete history of current and previous symptoms.

Contact your family doctor, local mental health center, or county health offices for treatment options.

✎ What's It Mean?

Major Depression: May occur several times in a person's life. It gets in the way of working, studying, sleeping, eating, and enjoying fun activities. Major depression can occur for the first time during the teenage years.

Dysthymia: A less severe type of depression that can be long lasting. It can keep a person from functioning well, feeling good, or experiencing joy. Dysthymia often starts during childhood or adolescence.

Bipolar Disorder: The least common type of depression, also called manic-depressive illness. The disorder can occur anytime from childhood to old age. A person who is bipolar will have cycles of mood changes, alternating between mania, a severe high, to depression, a severe low. Mania affects thinking, judgment, and social behavior in ways that can cause embarrassment and problems.

Source: Substance Abuse and Mental Health Services Administration, 2006.

event. Such events may include experiencing physical or sexual abuse; being a victim of or witnessing violence; or living through a disaster such as a bombing or hurricane. Young people with post-traumatic stress disorder experience the event over and over through strong memories, flashbacks, or other kinds of troublesome thoughts. As a result, they may try to avoid anything associated with the trauma. They also may overreact when startled or have difficulty sleeping.

Who is at risk?

Researchers have found that the basic temperament of young people may play a role in some childhood and adolescent anxiety disorders. For example, some children tend to be very shy and restrained in unfamiliar situations, a possible sign that they are at risk for developing an anxiety disorder. Research in this area is very complex, because children's fears often change as they age.

Researchers also suggest watching for signs of anxiety disorders when children are between the ages of six and eight. During this time, children generally grow less afraid of the dark and imaginary creatures and become more anxious about school performance and social relationships. An excessive amount of anxiety in children this age may be a warning sign for the development of anxiety disorders later in life.

♣ **It's A Fact!!**
How common are anxiety disorders?

Anxiety disorders are among the most common mental, emotional, and behavioral problems to occur during childhood and adolescence. About 13 of every 100 children and adolescents ages 9 to 17 experience some kind of anxiety disorder; girls are affected more than boys. About half of children and adolescents with anxiety disorders have a second anxiety disorder or other mental or behavioral disorder such as depression. In addition, anxiety disorders may co-exist with physical health conditions requiring treatment.

Source: Substance Abuse and Mental Health Services Administration, 2003.

Studies suggest that children or adolescents are more likely to have an anxiety disorder if they have a parent with anxiety disorders. However, the studies do not prove whether the disorders are caused by biology, environment, or both. More data are needed to clarify whether anxiety disorders can be inherited.

What help is available for young people with anxiety disorders?

Children and adolescents with anxiety disorders can benefit from a variety of treatments and services. Following an accurate diagnosis, possible treatments include the following:

- cognitive-behavioral treatment, in which young people learn to deal with fears by modifying the ways they think and behave

- relaxation techniques

- biofeedback (to control stress and muscle tension)

- family therapy

- parent training

- medication

While cognitive-behavioral approaches are effective in treating some anxiety disorders, medications work well with others. Some people with anxiety disorders benefit from a combination of these treatments. More research is needed to determine what treatments work best for the various types of anxiety disorders.

What can you do?

If you notice repeated symptoms of an anxiety disorder you should do the following:

- Talk with your health care provider. He or she can help to determine whether the symptoms are caused by an anxiety disorder or by some other condition and can also provide a referral to a mental health professional.

- Look for a mental health professional trained in working with children and adolescents, who has used cognitive-behavioral or behavior therapy and has prescribed medications for this disorder, or has co-operated with a physician who does.

You don't have to be hurt to experience PTSD—for some people, simply witnessing or being threatened with great physical harm is enough to trigger it. Events that can lead to PTSD involve feelings of helplessness, fear, or horror, and a sense that life or safety is in danger.

It's normal to be stressed out and anxious after going through something traumatic. Strong emotions, jitters, and trouble sleeping, eating, or concentrating may all be part of a normal and temporary reaction to an overwhelming event. So might frequent thoughts and images of what happened, nightmares, or fears. Getting the right care and support after a traumatic experience can help these symptoms run their course and subside in a few days or weeks and allow a person to move on.

But when a person has PTSD, the symptoms of a stress reaction are intense and last for longer than a month. For some people, the symptoms of PTSD begin soon after the trauma. Other people may have a delayed reaction that comes months—or even years—later. Delayed PTSD symptoms can be triggered by different things, such as the anniversary of an event or seeing someone who was involved in the situation.

What are the symptoms of PTSD?

Whether it occurs right after the trauma or later on, PTSD has certain characteristic symptoms. These include the following:

- **Reliving The Traumatic Event:** Many people with PTSD have nightmares, flashbacks, or disturbing mental images about the trauma.

- **Avoiding Reminders Of The Trauma:** People with PTSD may avoid people, places, or activities that remind them of the stressful event. They may also avoid talking about what happened.

- **Emotional Numbness:** Many people with PTSD feel detached or apart from others and describe feeling numb to some of the emotions they used to have. For example, loving or pleasure feelings may seem dulled. This

♣ It's A Fact!!
People who have little family or social support after a trauma, and those who have experienced past trauma, tend to be more vulnerable to posttraumatic stress disorder.

could be caused by the overproduction of certain chemicals that block sensation during extreme stress.

• **Hyperalertness:** People with PTSD may be easily startled, on edge, jumpy, irritable, or tense. This may be due to high levels of stress hormones in the body. Normally, these hormones are part of the body's healthy fight or flight reaction to danger or stress. In cases of PTSD, however, the levels of these stress hormones may remain elevated long after they're needed, so the person constantly feels on edge. Difficulty concentrating and trouble sleeping may also be part of this hyperalert state.

Who develops PTSD?

People of any age—kids, teens, and adults—can develop PTSD after facing an overwhelmingly frightening event that threatens life or safety. But not everyone who experiences a serious trauma develops PTSD. In fact, most people do not. Many recover from life-threatening traumas (after a normal reaction to the stressful event and the right support) without having a lasting problem. This ability to cope and bounce back is called resilience.

What makes some people more resilient to extremely stressful events when others have trouble coping? Researchers have found that certain things can help someone to be more resilient and to recover quicker from trauma. Everything from a person's belief in their ability to overcome problems to the types of hormones a person's body produces may play a role in resilience to stress.

Another factor in stress resilience is relationships. Having strong support from family and friends and getting counseling right after a traumatic event are two things that help.

The intensity or circumstances of a trauma can influence a person's vulnerability to PTSD, too. National disasters like the terrorist attacks of 9/11 or the Oklahoma City bombing can cause widespread anxiety and posttraumatic effects, even in people who didn't experience the trauma directly. These events can make people feel vulnerable and may trigger PTSD in some kids, teens, and adults.

How is PTSD treated?

Unfortunately PTSD often doesn't just go away on its own. Without treatment, some symptoms of PTSD can last for months or years, or they may come and go in waves. The right treatment and support, however, can help people of all ages to recover from PTSD.

Mental health professionals (such as psychologists, psychiatrists, and counselors) who specialize in treating anxiety problems are usually experienced in working with people who have PTSD. Therapy for PTSD may involve gradually talking it through in a safe environment and learning coping skills that help a person relieve anxiety, fear, or panic. These include relaxation techniques that help people with PTSD reset their stress response and techniques to resolve other problems, such as sleeping difficulties. Sometimes medications can help reduce symptoms of anxiety, panic, or depression in certain people.

Healing From Trauma

Sometimes people avoid seeking professional help because they're afraid that talking about an incident will bring back memories or feelings that are too painful. It can be difficult to talk about a traumatic event at first, but doing it in a safe environment with the help and support of a trained professional is the best way to ensure long-term healing. Working through the pain can help reduce symptoms like nightmares and flashbacks. It can also help people avoid potentially harmful behaviors and emotions, like extreme anger or self-injury.

☞ **Remember!!**

Posttraumatic stress disorder can be treated successfully. But if it's not treated it may continue for a long time. Some people learn that in the process of healing from trauma they discover strengths they didn't know they had. Others find that treatment helps them develop new insights into life and how to cope with other problems.

So how do you find the right therapist or counselor for you? The best way is to ask a parent or adult you trust for help. People who are close to you know you well and understand your needs. (Having a support system of family and friends is key to recovering from PTSD.) A doctor or school counselor may also be able to help you find a mental health professional who specializes in anxiety problems. And there are lots of resources available to help locate therapists in your area.

Turning to a professional for help in overcoming PTSD doesn't mean you're weak, and it doesn't mean you're crazy. PTSD is like any physical illness. The body's systems aren't working properly and treatment is needed to fix the problem. In the case of PTSD, the stress response system isn't switching off as it should; instead, it's constantly (or frequently) vigilant when it no longer needs to be. A therapist can help a person deal with the feelings of guilt, shame, or anger that may accompany PTSD—and discover inner strengths that can promote healing.

Chapter 37

Dissociative Disorders

Once considered rare and mysterious psychiatric curiosities, dissociative identity disorder (DID) (previously known as multiple personality disorder, or MPD) and other dissociative disorders are now understood to be fairly common effects of severe trauma in early childhood, most typically extreme, repeated physical, sexual, and/or emotional abuse.

Posttraumatic stress disorder (PTSD), widely accepted as a major mental illness affecting 8% of the general population in the United States, is closely related to dissociative disorders. In fact, 80–100% of people diagnosed with a dissociative disorder also have a secondary diagnosis of PTSD. The personal and societal cost of trauma disorders is extremely high. Recent research suggests the risk of suicide attempts among people with trauma disorders may be even higher than among people who have major depression. In addition, there is evidence that people with trauma disorders have higher rates of alcoholism, chronic medical illnesses, and abusiveness in succeeding generations.

About This Chapter: Information in this chapter is from "What Is a Dissociative Disorder?" © 1999, Sidran Institute. Reprinted with permission. Sidran Institute is a nonprofit organization that helps people understand, recover from, and treat traumatic stress, dissociative disorders, and co-occurring issues such as addictions, self-injury, and suicidality. Sidran develops and delivers education programming, resources for treatment, support, and self-help, community and professional collaboration projects, and publications about trauma and recovery. For more information about Sidran Institute, visit the website at www.sidran.org. Despite the older date of this document, the information presented is still appropriate for readers seeking to understand dissociative disorders.

What is dissociation?

Dissociation is a mental process, which produces a lack of connection in a person's thoughts, memories, feelings, actions, or sense of identity. During the period of time when a person is dissociating, certain information is not associated with other information as it normally would be. For example, during a traumatic experience, a person may dissociate the memory of the place and circumstances of the trauma from his ongoing memory, resulting in a temporary mental escape from the fear and pain of the trauma and, in some cases, a memory gap surrounding the experience. Because this process can produce changes in memory, people who frequently dissociate often find their senses of personal history and identity are affected.

Most clinicians believe that dissociation exists on a continuum of severity. This continuum reflects a wide range of experiences and/or symptoms. At one end are mild dissociative experiences common to most people, such as daydreaming, highway hypnosis, or "getting lost" in a book or movie, all of which involve "losing touch" with conscious awareness of one's immediate surroundings. At the other extreme is complex, chronic dissociation, such as in cases of dissociative disorders, which may result in serious impairment or inability to function. Some people with dissociative disorders can hold highly responsible jobs, contributing to society in a variety of professions, the arts, and public service—appearing to function normally to co-workers, neighbors, and others with whom they interact daily.

There is a great deal of overlap of symptoms and experiences among the various dissociative disorders, including DID. For the sake of clarity, this chapter will refer to dissociative disorders as a collective term. Individuals should seek help from qualified mental health providers to answer questions about their own particular circumstances and diagnoses.

How does a dissociative disorder develop?

When faced with overwhelmingly traumatic situations from which there is no physical escape, a child may resort to "going away" in his or her head. Children typically use this ability as an extremely effective defense against acute physical and emotional pain or anxious anticipation of that pain. By this dissociative process, thoughts, feelings, memories, and perceptions of the traumatic experiences can be separated off psychologically, allowing the child to function as if the trauma had not occurred.

Dissociative disorders are often referred to as a highly creative survival technique because they allow individuals enduring "hopeless" circumstances to preserve some areas of healthy functioning. Over time, however, for a child who has been repeatedly physically and sexually assaulted, defensive dissociation becomes reinforced and conditioned. Because the dissociative escape is so effective, children who are very practiced at it may automatically use it whenever they feel threatened or anxious—even if the anxiety-producing situation is not extreme or abusive.

Often, even after the traumatic circumstances are long past, the leftover pattern of defensive dissociation remains. Chronic defensive dissociation may lead to serious dysfunction in work, social, and daily activities.

Repeated dissociation may result in a series of separate entities, or mental states, which may eventually take on identities of their own. These entities may become the internal "personality states" of a DID system. Changing between these states of consciousness is often described as "switching."

What are the symptoms of a dissociative disorder?

People with dissociative disorders may experience any of the following: depression, mood swings, suicidal tendencies, sleep disorders (insomnia, night terrors, and sleep walking), panic attacks and phobias (flashbacks, reactions to stimuli or "triggers"), alcohol and drug abuse, compulsions and rituals, psychotic-like symptoms (including auditory and visual hallucinations), and eating disorders. In addition, individuals with dissociative disorders can experience headaches, amnesias, time loss, trances, and "out of body experiences." Some people with dissociative disorders have a tendency toward self-persecution, self-sabotage, and even violence (both self-inflicted and outwardly directed).

Who gets dissociative disorders?

The vast majority (as many as 98 to 99%) of individuals who develop dissociative disorders have documented histories of repetitive, overwhelming, and often life-threatening trauma at a sensitive developmental stage of childhood (usually before the age of nine), and they may possess an inherited biological predisposition for dissociation. In our culture, the most frequent precursor to dissociative disorders is extreme physical, emotional, and sexual abuse in childhood, but survivors of other kinds of trauma in childhood (such as natural disasters, invasive medical procedures, war, kidnapping, and torture) have also reacted by developing dissociative disorders.

♣ **It's A Fact!!**
In our culture, the most frequent precursor to dissociative disorders is extreme physical, emotional, and sexual abuse in childhood.

Current research shows that DID may affect 1% of the general population and perhaps as many as 5–20% of people in psychiatric hospitals, many of whom have received other diagnoses. The incidence rates are even higher among sexual abuse survivors and individuals with chemical dependencies. These statistics put dissociative disorders in the same category as schizophrenia, depression, and anxiety, as one of the four major mental health problems today.

Most current literature shows that dissociative disorders are recognized primarily among females. The latest research, however, indicates that the disorders may be equally prevalent (but less frequently diagnosed) among the male population. Men with dissociative disorders are most likely to be in treatment for other mental illnesses or drug and alcohol abuse, or they may be incarcerated.

Why are dissociative disorders often misdiagnosed?

Dissociative disorders survivors often spend years living with misdiagnoses, consequently floundering within the mental health system. They change from therapist to therapist and from medication to medication, getting treatment for symptoms but making little or no actual progress. Research has documented that on average, people with dissociative disorders have spent seven years in the mental health system prior to accurate diagnosis. This is common because the list of symptoms that cause a person with a dissociative disorder to seek treatment is very similar to those of many other psychiatric diagnoses.

Do people actually have "multiple personalities"?

Yes and no. One of the reasons for the decision by the psychiatric community to change the disorder's name from multiple personality disorder to dissociative identity disorder is that "multiple personalities" is somewhat of a misleading term. A person diagnosed with DID feels as if she has within her two or more entities, or personality states, each with its own independent way of relating, perceiving, thinking, and remembering about herself and her life. If two or more of these entities take control of the person's behavior at a given time, a diagnosis of DID can be made. These entities previously were often called "personalities," even though the term did not accurately reflect the common definition of the word as the total aspect of our psychological makeup. Other terms often used by therapists and survivors to describe these entities are: "alternate personalities," "alters," "parts," "states of consciousness," "ego states," and "identities." It is important to keep in mind that although these alternate states may appear to be very different, they are all manifestations of a single person.

Can dissociative disorders be cured?

✦ It's A Fact!!

Many people who are diagnosed with dissociative disorders also have secondary diagnoses of depression, anxiety, or panic disorders.

Yes. Dissociative disorders are highly responsive to individual psychotherapy, or "talk therapy," as well as to a range of other treatment modalities including medications, hypnotherapy, and adjunctive therapies such as art or movement therapy. In fact, among comparably severe psychiatric disorders, dissociative disorders may be the condition that carries the best prognosis if proper treatment is undertaken and completed. The course of treatment is long-term, intensive, and invariably painful, as it generally involves remembering and reclaiming the dissociated traumatic experiences. Nevertheless, individuals with dissociative disorders have been successfully treated by therapists of all professional backgrounds working in a variety of settings.

Chapter 38

How Can Domestic Violence
And Abuse Be Prevented And Treated?

How can a woman safely leave an abusive relationship and protect herself from further abuse? Most women cannot simply leave their homes, their jobs, their children's schools, their friends, and their relatives to escape their abuser. They depend upon police to enforce the law against physical abuse. Yet, police cannot act until a restraining order is violated or until some physical harm again befalls the woman.

If you are a victim of domestic violence, you may believe that it's easier to stay with your abuser than to try to leave and risk retaliation. However, there are many things you can do to protect yourself while getting out of an abusive situation, and there are people waiting to help.

How can I get help as a victim of domestic abuse or domestic violence?

For Emergency Help: Call 911 if you are in immediate danger of domestic violence or have already been hurt.

About This Chapter: "Domestic Violence and Abuse: Help, Treatment, Intervention, and Prevention," by Tina de Benedictis, Ph.D., Jaelline Jaffe, Ph.D., and Jeanne Segal, Ph.D., reprinted with permission from http://www.helpguide.org/mental/domestic_violence_abuse _help_treatment_prevention.htm. © 2007 Helpguide.org. All rights reserved. Helpguide provides a detailed list of related references for this article, including links to information from other websites. For a complete list of Helpguide's current resources related to help for domestic abuse and domestic violence, visit www.helpguide.org.

For Advice And Support: Call the National Domestic Violence Hotline at 1-800-799-7233 (SAFE). Additional contacts for the National Domestic Violence Hotline:

- Help via e-mail: ndvh@ndvh.org
- For the hearing-impaired: 1-800-787-3224 (TTY)
- For the deaf: deafhelp@ndvh.org

For A Safe Place To Stay: Call your state's branch of the National Coalition Against Domestic Violence if you need a shelter from domestic violence. To find your state's hotline number, go to the State Coalition List at http://www.ncadv.org/resources/StateCoalitionList_73.html.

What can I do to protect myself from domestic violence?

If you live with someone who abuses you, you need to protect yourself for the long term. If someone is stalking you, and you have a feeling that you might get hurt, trust your instincts and protect yourself.

You are in extra danger if your abuser or stalker talks about murder or suicide. You are also in particular danger if you are thinking of leaving the relationship. Because of the risk of being seriously hurt or killed when leaving an abusive relationship, it is important to develop a safe plan for departure.

- Take all threats seriously.

- Contact a domestic violence hotline to plan for your safe future. People who are staffing the phones or e-mail can advise you on how to protect yourself, refer you to other services and shelters, and inform you about local laws and restraining orders.

- Develop a safety plan that specifies who will be with you when you need companionship and protection. Also plan for safety in your workplace or at your school.

- Call people who are willing to help you and tell them how they can help to protect you now and in the future.

- If you have been abused in front of others, ask witnesses to write down what they saw.

- Contact the police if your abuser has broken a law or even if you just think they might have broken a law. Assaulting you or stealing or destroying your property is a crime.

- Consider getting a restraining order or protective order to keep your spouse or intimate partner away from you.

- Learn self-defense to protect yourself.

How useful is a restraining order or protection order against domestic violence?

A restraining order has no force behind it, in and of itself. It is just a piece of paper. The police can enforce the order only if someone violates it, and then only if someone reports the violation. This means that you must be endangered in some way for the police to step in.

If you are the victim of stalking or abuse, you need to carefully research how restraining orders or protection orders are enforced in your neighborhood. Find out if the violator will just be given a citation or if they will actually be taken to jail. If the police simply talk to the violator or give a citation, the abuser may reason that the police will do nothing and feel empowered to pursue you further. Or the abuser may become angry and retaliate.

> ✔ **Quick Tip**
>
> Do not feel falsely secure with a restraining order. You are not necessarily safe if you have a restraining order or protection order. The stalker or abuser may ignore it, and the police may do nothing to enforce it.
>
> To learn about restraining orders in your area, call 1-800-799-7233 (SAFE) or contact your state's Domestic Violence Coalition.

I am afraid to seek help or to leave my partner. How can I get help safely?

If you are afraid to seek help because you think your partner will retaliate if they find out, you need to be especially careful. You may be right. Following are some ways to keep safe as you seek help.

Seeking Help By Phone: When you seek help by phone, use a corded phone, rather than a cordless phone or cell phone and one of the following:

- a prepaid phone card
- a friend's telephone charge card
- coins
- call collect

If you use your own home phone or telephone charge card, the phone numbers that you called will be listed on the monthly bill that is sent to your home. Some abusers wish to control your every move, and your seeking help may be interpreted as an affront. Additionally, you don't want your abuser to be able to track you down by the phone numbers of places you have called for help.

Online Help: If you seek help online, you are safest if you use a computer outside of your home. You can use a computer at a domestic violence shelter or agency, at work, at a friend's house, at a library, or at a community center.

It is almost impossible to clear a computer of evidence of the websites that you have visited, unless you know a lot about internet browsers and about your own computer. Read "Internet Security" at http://www.womenslaw.org/internet.htm for instructions for covering your online tracks and e-mail history but be wary of leaving traces that your abuser might find.

Going To A Domestic Violence Shelter Or Women's Refuge: If you go to a domestic violence shelter or women's refuge, you do not have to give identifying information about yourself, even if asked. Leaving identifying information at a shelter could be a problem if your abuser gained access to it.

In addition, you can get a mailing address that keeps your new home address confidential. For example, the State of California has a mail-forwarding service called Safe at Home. Ask the National Domestic Violence Hotline for help in finding a service that will confidentially forward your mail to your real home address.

What is a domestic violence shelter?

A domestic violence shelter is a building or set of apartments where victims of domestic violence can go to seek refuge from their abusers. A family might also host a victim of domestic violence in their home in return for a small stipend from the domestic violence agency. The location of the shelter is kept confidential from the public, and each visitor must also keep the location private. Basic living needs will be provided for by the domestic violence agency for a short time.

The length of time that the victim can stay at the shelter is limited, but there are usually resources to help victims find permanent homes. Shelters are primarily for women, as the number of men who are physically endangered by a woman is limited. Shelters generally have room for mothers and their children.

What kind of psychological help is available for me as a survivor of domestic abuse?

If you are a survivor of domestic violence, you need to get support in the form of counseling or therapy. The scars of domestic abuse are usually deeper than those from post-traumatic-stress disorder (PTSD). A lifetime of abuse leaves a different kind of scar than short-lived trauma. Brief counseling is usually not enough.

How do I report suspected domestic abuse?

Reporting suspected domestic abuse is important. If you're afraid of getting involved, remember that the report is confidential and everything possible will be done to protect your privacy. You do not have to give your name, and your

---

✔ **Quick Tip**

To be referred for counseling, contact:

- The National Domestic Violence Hotline: 1-800-799-7233 or ndvh@ndvh.org

- The National Coalition Against Domestic Violence: State Coalition List at http://www.ncadv.org/resources/StateCoalitionList_73.html

suspicions will be investigated before anyone is taken into custody. Most important, you can protect the victim from further harm by calling for help.

Call 911 or the police in your community if you suspect a case of domestic violence.

In the workplace, it is important that human resources personnel, managers, and employees know how to help victims of domestic abuse. Contact your Human Resources department if you suspect domestic violence. To learn more, visit "Strategic Employer Responses to Domestic Violence" at http:// endabuse.org/workplace/.

How do I get help if I am an abuser, or if I think I may abuse my spouse or intimate partner?

If you want to get help for someone you have just hurt, call 911. If you need to talk because you have just hurt someone or think you are about to hurt someone, call the National Domestic Violence Hotline at 1-800-799-7233.

You can get help if you are an abuser. The hotline can recommend programs to support you if you want to escape the cycle of violence. Available resources include the following:

- individual counseling

- group counseling

- batterer treatment programs

How can domestic violence and abuse be prevented or treated?

Treatment Programs: It has been difficult to craft programs that successfully help abusers or potential abusers stop the cycle of domestic violence. There has been greater success in developing programs that criminalize domestic violence or offer shelter and support to victims of domestic abuse. Initial treatment programs for abusers focused on anger management, but research indicates that anger management is not the problem. Most abusers can control their anger toward other people or in public. But they feel justified in aiming their anger toward their intimate partner at home. Thus, the current focus is on changing the abuser's attitude toward women. For more information, check out Treatment for Abusers at http://www.edvp.org/AboutDV/forabusers.htm.

Intervention In Childhood And During The Teen Years: Children who grow up in violent households are likely to be abusive as adults. However, this cycle of domestic violence can be broken. Education and intervention for children and teenagers is the most important place to start. To help children and teens at risk for becoming violent as adults, we must prevent further exposure to domestic violence and teach them nonviolent responses to stress.

Education: Education is key in preventing domestic abuse. Key issues include raising awareness about domestic violence, letting people know that domestic violence is a crime and that it will be punished, training medical professionals and counselors to recognize signs of abuse and to take action, and educating victims about their rights and how to get help.

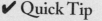

✔ Quick Tip

To learn how to build safe, intimate love relationships see Helpguide's "Building and Preserving Joy and Excitement in Adult Relationships" at http://www.helpguide.org/mental/improve_relationships.htm.

Chapter 39

When Parents Fight

Chances are you've had an argument or twenty with your parents recently—about clothes, homework, friends, curfew—pretty much anything. But what's going on when your parents fight with each other?

You may be a little relieved that, for once, you're not the one arguing with a parent. But most people worry when they hear their parents argue.

It's normal for parents to disagree and argue from time to time. They might disagree about important things like their careers, finances, or major family decisions. They might even disagree about little things that don't seem important at all—like what's for dinner or what time someone gets home.

Sometimes parents stay levelheaded when they disagree, and they allow each other a chance to listen and to talk. But many times when parents disagree, they argue.

What Does It Mean When Parents Fight?

When your parents are fighting, thoughts might start rushing around in your head: Why are they shouting at each other? Does this mean they don't love each other anymore? Are they going to get a divorce?

About This Chapter: This information was provided by TeensHealth, one of the largest resources online for medically reviewed health information written for teens, kids, and parents. For more articles like this one, visit www.TeensHealth.org, or www.KidsHealth.org. © 2006 The Nemours Foundation.

It can be easy to jump to conclusions when you hear parents argue. But most of the time, arguments are just a way to let off steam when parents have a bad day, don't feel well, or are under a lot of stress—kind of like when you argue with them.

Like you, when your parents get upset with each other they might yell, cry, or say things they don't really mean. Most people lose their cool now and then. So if your parents are fighting, don't always assume it means the worst.

It's OK For Parents To Argue Sometimes

It's natural for people to have different opinions, feelings, or approaches to things. Talking about these differences is a first step in working toward a mutually agreeable solution. It's important for people in a family to be able to tell each other how they feel and what they think, even when they disagree.

Sometimes parents can feel so strongly about their differences that it may lead to arguments. Most of the time, these arguments are over quickly, parents apologize and make up, and the family settles back into its usual routine.

When Parents' Fighting Goes Too Far

But sometimes when parents fight, there's too much yelling and screaming, name calling, and too many harsh things said. Although some parents may do this, it's not OK to treat people in the family with disrespect, use degrading or insulting language, or yell and scream at them.

Sometimes parents' fighting really goes too far, and includes pushing and shoving, throwing things, or hitting. Even if one parent is not physically injured, an argument has gone too far when one parent uses threats to try to control the other through fear. Examples include if a parent does the following:

- threatens to injure himself or herself
- threatens to commit suicide
- threatens to leave the other parent
- threatens to report the other parent to welfare
- destroys the other's property

These things are never OK. When fights get physical or involve threats, the people fighting need to learn to get their anger under control.

What About You?

It's hard for most people to hear their parents yelling at each other. Seeing them upset and out of control can throw you off—aren't parents supposed to be the calm, composed, and mature ones in the family? How much it bothers you might depend on how often it happens, how loud or intense things get, or whether parents argue in front of other people.

You might worry more about one parent or the other during an argument. It's natural to worry that a parent may feel especially hurt by what the other parent says. Or maybe you worry that one parent could become angry enough to lose control. Should you be worried that someone might get physically hurt? With all this extra mental and emotional stress, you may get a stomachache or want to go to your room and cry. It's understandable to feel this way when there's conflict around you.

> **☞ Remember!!**
>
> If your parents are arguing about you, this can be especially upsetting. Lots of people in this situation might mistakenly think the argument is their fault. But your parents' arguments are never your fault.

If your parents' fighting really bothers you, you might find it hard to sleep or go to school. If this is the case, try talking to one or both of your parents about their behavior. They may not even realize how upset you are until you tell them how their arguments affect you.

If you or someone you know lives in a family where the fighting goes too far, let someone else know what's going on. Talking to other relatives, a teacher, a school counselor, or any adult you trust about the fighting can be helpful. Sometimes parents who fight can get so out of control that they hurt each other or other family members. If this happens, letting someone else know will allow the family to be helped and protected from such harmful fighting.

Family members can learn to listen to each other and talk about feelings and differences without yelling and screaming. They can get help with problem fighting from counselors and therapists. Though it may take some work, time, and practice, people in families can always learn to get along better.

Happy, Healthy Families

If your family argues from time to time, try not to sweat it: No family is perfect. Even in the happiest home, problems pop up and people argue. Usually the family members involved get what's bothering them out in the open and talk about it. Hopefully, they can reach some compromise or agreement. Everyone feels better and life can get back to normal.

Being part of a family means everyone pitches in and tries to make life better for each other. Arguments happen and that's OK. But with love, understanding, and some work, families can solve almost any problem.

Chapter 40

What You Can Do To Help Stop Teen Violence

Start A School Crime Watch

What is a school crime watch?

Based on the Neighborhood Watch concept, a school crime watch helps youth watch out for each other to make the entire school area safer and more enjoyable. The school crime watch is a student-led effort that helps youth take a share of responsibility for their school community.

Youth who participate in a school crime watch learn how to keep from becoming victims. They also learn the best ways to report suspicious activities or arguments between students before they turn into fights or other disturbances.

About This Chapter: Information in this chapter under the heading "Start A School Crime Watch" is from "Stand Up and Start a School Crime Watch!" *Youth in action*, Number 03, December 1998, Office of Juvenile Justice and Delinquency Prevention, Office of Justice Programs, U.S. Department of Justice; http://www.ncjrs.gov/pdffiles/ 94601.pdf; accessed January 2007. Text under the heading "Arts And Performances For Prevention" is from "What Are Arts and Performances for Prevention?" *Youth in action*, Number 11, December 1999, Office of Juvenile Justice and Delinquency Prevention, Office of Justice Programs, U.S. Department of Justice; http://www.ncjrs.gov/html/ ojjdp/youthbulletin/9912_1/art1.html; accessed January 2007. Despite the older date of these documents, the information presented is still appropriate for readers seeking to understand what they can do to help stop teen violence.

How does a school crime watch prevent or reduce crime?

An organized school crime watch program provides youth with a focus, a source of reliable information, and a core of committed youth who will make crime prevention a priority in the school community. The crime watch reminds everyone of prevention strategies they can use and helps build schoolwide resistance to criminal activities.

Having such a group on campus says, "Crime is not tolerated here" and provides a way for students to respond to crime incidents and issues.

What does it take to start a school crime watch?

It only takes one person to start a school crime watch. A concerned adult might talk to students about the idea. A group of students may be fed up with bullying or intimidation. An especially violent incident at or near school might have everyone wondering how to stop violence from happening again. A youth might realize that crime, though not a major threat, needs to be addressed before it becomes a problem.

♣ **It's A Fact!!**
At Carol City High School in Miami, Florida, crime dropped 45 percent within a year of the beginning of a school crime watch program.

Source: Excerpted from "Stand Up and Start a School Crime Watch!" *Youth in action*, Number 03, December 1998, U.S. Department of Justice.

Take The Plunge: Whatever your reason may be for wanting to start a school crime watch, the first task is to gather a group of youth willing to work together to bring the entire student body into a "crime watch" way of life. This group should represent the diversity of the school community. Try to involve as many people as possible. Reach beyond your immediate circle of friends for volunteers.

Getting the entire student body to watch out, help out, and report crime is an ongoing task that will not happen overnight. Your group will need to do the following:

- Find out which crimes (e.g., vandalism, assault, theft, substance abuse) are most common at school.

- Determine what other issues you want to address (e.g., arguments, smoking, weapons, bullying).

- Decide which prevention strategies could prove the most effective.

Much of the information you will need can be obtained from guidance counselors, school security staff, city or county school officials, local law enforcement, and students themselves.

Develop Partnerships: Starting up the program will require a close working relationship with school authorities, including the principal, other officials charged with school security, and local law enforcement (especially the crime prevention staff). Your group should develop a close partnership with these officials and keep them informed of your ideas, plans, and activities.

All partners involved in the crime watch should agree on its mission and objectives. As a group, you may want to discuss whether a student patrol should be incorporated into the crime watch. Representatives of all partner organizations (e.g., school officials and local law enforcement) should be present at the group's first meeting and should be notified of all developments and progress.

Sponsor A Program Kickoff: Another key issue is deciding how to kick off the program. One way to do this is to plan a school-wide meeting to introduce the program and its mission. This could be a school assembly held during class time or an after school meeting. You will need to discuss this with your school administrators. Advertise the program's kickoff widely through the school newspaper, public address (PA) announcements, fliers, posters, e-mail, and websites. The more people who know of and attend the kickoff event, the better.

The kickoff event is also an excellent recruiting ground for bringing in more volunteers. Make the kickoff meeting exciting; use music, skits—maybe even a light show. Introduce the program in such a way that everyone will want to be involved.

Educate other students, faculty, and staff on the roles and purposes of the school crime watch, and give them helpful prevention tips relevant to problems they are facing. In addition, teach them how and what to report, and encourage them to view themselves as key members of the effort.

Provide Training: Once you have gathered volunteers to participate in your school crime watch and decided on your specific activities, you will need to provide some training. Training will make sure that all participants understand the goals and objectives of your project, that they have the skills necessary to perform tasks, and that they know how to handle problems. Training also builds teamwork among your volunteers and develops the skills needed for the success of your project. You will need to plan such details as the following:

- when and where a training session will take place

- contents and procedures of a training session

- what, if any, additional materials will be needed

You may also need to enlist the help of such professionals as law enforcement officers, victim assistance professionals, school security staff, trainers from corporations, lawyers, and community volunteer agencies.

Be sure each specific part of the training is planned. This will do much to ensure the success of your effort. Professional trainers know that preparation and organization are 80 percent of good training.

What are some possible school crime watch activities?

Student Patrol Program: A student patrol can be a powerful component of a school crime watch. These groups go beyond traffic safety patrol programs. They look for and report signs of crime and help keep crime off campuses. This moves the program from an informational and teaching posture to one of action.

Patrol activities include monitoring halls and parking lots between classes and during lunch. This alone can reduce the number of crime-related incidents. Recognize, however, that if the patrol is not accepted by a majority of students, it can easily be seen as a group of "snitches."

♣ **It's A Fact!!**

In schools with active patrols, crime has dropped 20 to 75 percent.

Source: Excerpted from "Stand Up and Start a School Crime Watch!"
Youth in action, Number 03, December 1998, U.S. Department
of Justice.

Anonymous Reporting System: Another school crime watch activity is setting up an anonymous reporting system. A reporting system is critical to the success of a school crime watch program. Students should report crime or incidents because they are serious issues, not because they want to get someone they do not like into trouble. If an incident is not reported, it might escalate into a dangerous situation for the students involved.

Reporting should be done on an anonymous basis, and all crime watch reports should be kept confidential. Such a reporting system can produce tips on areas to watch on the school grounds and reveal other issues of concern to students.

Other Activities: Student crime watch programs can perform a number of other activities to promote the overall health of the school. These include the following:

• hosting drug- and alcohol-free parties

• sponsoring crime prevention fairs

• working with local elementary schools on child safety issues

• writing a column about crime prevention for your local or school newspaper

• presenting daily or weekly crime prevention tips over the PA system during morning announcements

• teaching drug prevention, personal safety, and conflict resolution to peers and younger students

• organizing school cleanups

What does it take to keep a school crime watch going?

A monthly meeting keeps the momentum and energy building for your school crime watch program and keeps you focused on your goals. At these meetings, the group can plan new activities and track the progress of ongoing activities such as the student patrol.

Make a calendar of crime watch events and distribute it at school. This allows all students to be informed of upcoming activities. The calendar can also list other events and act as a resource for prevention news.

You may want to purchase T-shirts or baseball caps that identify the school crime watch participants and the student patrol. This will build pride in your program and strengthen its identity as an important part of school life.

Suggest to school officials that information on school safety and on the crime watch program be distributed at the orientation for new students. Members of the school crime watch could present the information, give a brief description of the program, and recruit volunteers.

What are some of the challenges of a school crime watch?

Maintaining Interest: In any crime watch program, maintaining interest and excitement is always a challenge. People do not want to simply stand around and watch for trouble to happen; they want to do something. That is why an active, school-linked program is important.

Excluding certain social groups in your school, even unintentionally, is a threat to the success of a school crime watch. It is not just for athletes, students in school government, or high achievers.

♣ It's A Fact!!

A school crime watch must be seen to belong to everyone, not just one or two selected groups.

Source: Excerpted from "Stand Up and Start a School Crime Watch!" *Youth in action*, Number 03, December 1998, U.S. Department of Justice.

> ## ✦ It's A Fact!!
> Running a successful crime watch requires getting participants to understand they are not vigilantes. The term is "watch," not "capture." Students should report trouble quickly, not seek to catch the offenders themselves.
>
> Source: Excerpted from "Stand Up and Start a School Crime Watch!" *Youth in action*, Number 03, December 1998, U.S. Department of Justice.

Maintaining Privacy: Another challenge is maintaining the privacy of any reporting system. Crime watch members should understand that sharing the sources of reports with those outside the project can jeopardize the entire program and cannot be tolerated. Stress that if students find out who reported them, it could become dangerous for those doing the reporting. It could also undermine the integrity of the program and influence students to not participate in the program. Nobody wants to put themselves or others in dangerous situations.

What are some of the rewards of a school crime watch?

Active school crime watch programs have helped reduce violence, the presence of guns, drug use, and many other crime-related activities in schools across the country. Schools where these programs are in place report a happier student body and safer campuses with more school spirit. Students and staff feel free to enjoy the school setting instead of fearing crime on campus. Students actively involved in the program gain leadership skills and an understanding of crime prevention and community organizing.

How can a school crime watch program be evaluated?

Evaluating your project can help you learn whether it has met its goals, but only if you decide up front what you want to evaluate and how you will go about doing so. The purpose of conducting an evaluation is to answer practical questions of decision makers and program implementers who want to know whether to continue a program, extend it to other sites, modify it, or close it down. You will want to be able to show that your project does one or all of the following:

- reduces crime

- reduces fear of crime

- is cost effective

- has a lasting impact

- attracts support and resources

- makes people feel safe and better about being in their school or community

The best way to start evaluating your project is to reflect on your original goals:

- Was crime reduced in and around your school?

- Did you reach all the people in the school community you intended to?

- Did the message of your project reach other youth? Did they learn what you were trying to teach them?

- Are young people more aware of their surroundings while at school?

Be sure to include an evaluation step in your overall plan. Ask yourself what you can do better to reach your goals, to involve more people in your project, and to spread your message to a wider audience. Then, make adjustments to your activities to strengthen your project.

The most tangible way to evaluate a school crime watch program is to track the number of incidents or crimes reported. If there is a decrease in incidents while the program is active, the school crime watch can be considered successful, especially if similar schools without crime watches have seen crime increase or stay the same. Surveys about how safe people feel at school can also provide important evaluation data. Tabulating the number of participants, events sponsored, and their success, and testing the knowledge of crime prevention among students and staff, are also good evaluation measures.

Learning to evaluate the things you do is a good skill and one you can apply to all aspects of your life.

Arts And Performances For Prevention

What are arts and performances for prevention?

Through music, drama, dance, and visual arts, youth can draw attention to problems in their communities, educate others on the benefits of crime prevention, and suggest ways to prevent crime. Arts and performances for prevention may take many forms, from 10-minute skits to full-length plays, from rap to opera, from posters to sculptures, from murals to musical compositions. Youth across the nation have produced videos and photo essays, designed T-shirts and ceramics, played saxophones and violins, and danced ballet and modern jazz—all to promote the prevention of crime and violence.

How do arts and performances prevent or reduce crime?

Because they reach a wide audience, arts and performances are effective ways to prevent or reduce crime. By reaching new audiences with each performance or display, arts and performances increase awareness and refresh anti-crime messages for those who may have heard but forgotten them. They also communicate messages in multiple ways to emphasize key ideas, allowing youth to use their artistic, musical, dramatic, and other talents to deliver vital information to the community.

By allowing youth to use their creative talents, arts and performances help youth develop a sense of identity, independence, discipline, and self-worth. They also help prevent or reduce crime and violence among the young artists and performers involved.

What does it take to start?

At the heart of any art or performance activity is the talent of the young people involved. Your group's talents should support the goal of the performance, product, or show. Depending on the type of performance planned, your group may need musicians, dancers, set builders, sculptors, actors, stagehands, watercolorists, costume designers, makeup artists, or poets. Your group members should also agree on a central message—for example, that they want to fight drug abuse, reduce hate crimes, or discourage violence. An adult may suggest an idea, but it is the young group members' commitment and talent that will communicate the message to the community.

As with any crime prevention project, the best way to ensure your group's success is by planning well. These three steps can help you get started:

1. Identify your audience and message. Your group needs to decide whom it will reach and what it will say. Is the target audience young people? Adults? Or maybe a group of mixed ages? Identifying the age group of the audience will help you decide how to present your message. A modern dance performance presented to young children, for example, may need to be narrated and have more frequent intermissions than one performed for adults.

♣ **It's A Fact!!**

According to research, students who participate in band, orchestra, chorus, or drama are significantly less likely than non-participants to drop out of school, be arrested, use drugs, or engage in binge drinking.

Source: Excerpted from "Arts and Performances for Prevention" *Youth in action*, Number 11, December 1999, U.S. Department of Justice.

At the same time, consider what subject or message your group wants to emphasize. Do you want to present one general idea such as "Stop the Violence"? Or do you want to relay specific information to the audience such as how to prevent date rape? If you want to present only one theme, you could sponsor an exhibit of different paintings on that theme at your school or community center. Focusing on art dealing with one subject may make a stronger statement than including dozens of paintings on dozens of different crime prevention themes. If you decide to concentrate on a more complex issue such as date rape or substance abuse, consider doing a play or skit.

2. Identify your needs and available resources. After you decide on the audience and message, you will have to determine what you will need for your activity. Will you need costumes, performance or exhibit space, rehearsal space, materials for props, music, a performance program, and a way to publicize the event?

Some of these items may be donated by schools, churches, universities, or businesses. Use your school's public address system or school newspaper to ask for donations. You may also be able to obtain discounts or sponsorship from local businesses. Let them know that donations may result in excellent publicity. A local printing shop may be willing to give you a discount on printing if you agree to provide free advertising in your program.

Although your arts and performances program is an activity led and performed by youth, you will probably need assistance from one or more adults. Recruit at least one adult to be your sponsor or adviser. Community members with experience in the arts—drama teachers, parents, neighbors, and local community theater actors—may donate special talent or agree to act as advisers, coaches, or directors. It is important to make a thorough list of your project's needs right away and to keep adding to it as new needs arise.

3. Develop a schedule. A third major task is developing a realistic schedule for your presentation or display. In creating a schedule, consider such things as whether you are presenting a published work or bringing a brand new play or song to the stage. A new work may take longer to produce but may be worth the wait. Likewise, if your artists do not paint well under pressure, leave plenty of time in your schedule to allow them to work effectively.

You will also need to do the following:

- Find out when space is available.

- Assess how long it will take to make costumes.

- Determine how long it will take to construct and paint sets and collect or make props.

Thinking about and planning for these factors will help you develop an overall timeline and allow you to be ready for your performance or display.

What does it take to keep it going?

Maintaining community support is perhaps the greatest challenge for keeping arts and performances programs alive. Although most program funding comes from local sources, identifying and generating new resources both within and outside your community is vital. You may be able to establish partnerships with community centers and other youth organizations. Through such partnerships, you may be able to form advisory boards or committees that will coordinate a set number of performances or displays each year.

Many arts and performances programs for youth operate in partnership with high schools, universities, youth organizations, churches, businesses, community theaters, and health agencies. Community-based arts agencies may be excellent sources of information and support. Investigate whether any organizations in your community would be interested in supporting a youth program that harnesses the power of artistic communication to prevent crime. Talk to teachers, local business owners, civic groups, local government agencies, and practicing artists to see if they would be willing to help.

What are some of the challenges?

Experience has shown that many arts and performances initiatives are unable to survive without sustained support and new resources. To meet this challenge, program leaders need to identify funding sources on an ongoing basis. State funding, business support, or local foundation funding is sometimes available, but identifying funding sources takes time and requires research. Successful grant applicants must show a clear mission, measurable goals, and an independent evaluation of their efforts.

In addition to financial challenges, your arts and performances will face an ongoing need for rehearsal, performance, or display space. If possible, work out an agreement with a local school, church, library, or other organization to use necessary space. Recruiting artists, performers, group members, and other volunteers is

> ✔ **Quick Tip**
>
> Another way to maintain an arts and performances program is by sharing resources with other similar programs. For example, your members may be able to learn from other groups or train at their centers. Mentorship programs and performance exchanges help to create networks and enrich existing programs. Fostering communication and collaboration among centers also strengthens each program.
>
> Source: Excerpted from "Arts and Performances for Prevention" *Youth in action*, Number 11, December 1999, U.S. Department of Justice.

another challenge facing arts and performances programs. As members graduate from high school, move away from the area, or shift interests, your group will need to devote time and energy to recruiting new and talented members.

What are some of the rewards?

Many benefits result from using arts and performances to help prevent crime. In addition to the satisfaction of creating or performing, you will have the pleasure of knowing that you have communicated about a subject of vital interest to your community. As a result of your work, young children may learn new ways to settle arguments peacefully, adults may learn how to help establish a crime-free community, and your peers may realize that they need help with personal problems or recognize the importance of taking a stand against drugs.

Because dance, music, photography, and other arts transcend language, they often help to bridge cultural, racial, and ethnic barriers. A photography exhibit, play, or recital can also generate real enthusiasm for your group members' abilities and provide much-deserved recognition from adults and your peers. After all of your work, you will see that you have had a good time and probably made or strengthened friendships.

How can your project be evaluated?

Evaluating your project allows you to find out whether it has met its goals. Evaluation works, however, only if you decide up front what you want to evaluate and how you will do so. The purpose of conducting an evaluation is to answer practical questions of decision makers and program implementers who want to know whether to continue a program, extend it to other sites, modify it, or close it down. When evaluating your group's performance or display, you will want to show that your project does one or all of the following:

- engages the talent of local youth in promoting a key crime prevention message

- provides opportunities for youth to use and develop artistic ability

- educates and raises community members' awareness of the problems or issues that your group chose to address

- uses creative expression to transcend language and cultural barriers

You can evaluate your effort in two ways. First, you can assess your audience's response. Did the audience enjoy the performance? Did it understand the anti-crime or anti-drug message you intended to convey? Applause, encores, and positive comments in guest books are good indicators of audience enjoyment. A survey asking audience members about the theme(s) of a performance or display also can help you check on their learning. In working with children, you may want to ask simple questions to probe their understanding and see how well they are able to apply your message to their own lives.

Second, you can consider your program's effect on the group's participants. Are they more confident? Have they learned valuable information about crime and drug abuse prevention? Survey group participants and those involved in developing your performance or display; ask them how the program helped them and exactly what they learned.

In evaluating your arts and performances program, also consider whether, and how, it meets the following more general crime prevention goals:

- reduces crime or fear of crime in your community

- is cost-effective

- has a lasting impact

- attracts support and resources

- makes people feel safer and more positive about being a member of your school or community

Learning to evaluate the things you do is a good skill and one you can apply to all aspects of your life.

Chapter 41

After-School Programs Help Prevent Teen Violence

The hours immediately after school can be a dangerous time for teenagers. During these hours, teens are more likely to commit violent crimes and to be the victims of violence than at any other time in the day or night. While many teens use this time productively, others spend these hours engaging in risky behaviors that can harm their future prospects. Fortunately, increasing numbers of teens are staying safe and using this time to learn, grow, explore, and make a difference by participating in after-school programs.

The After-School Hours Can Be Dangerous For Teens

During after-school hours, children and teens are more likely to become victims of violent crime than at other times. For teens ages 12 to 17, this risk peaks at 3 o'clock in the afternoon, the end of the school day.

Violence by teens peaks in the hours immediately after school. While crimes by adults peak at 11 o'clock at night, violent crimes by juveniles peak between 3 p.m. and 4 p.m. on school days.

Many teens get involved in dangerous and risky activities during the after-school hours. Millions of children and teens spend the hours after school

About This Chapter: Information in this chapter is from "After-School Programs," National Youth Violence Prevention Resource Center, 2002.

unsupervised. Unfortunately, children and teens that are not supervised by adults, or involved in structured activities after school, are much more likely to do the following:

- use alcohol, drugs, and tobacco

- receive poor grades and skip or drop out of school

- engage in risky sexual activity

- get arrested

- carry and use weapons

> ♣ **It's A Fact!!**
> Juveniles injure more victims in the hours around the close of school than any other time of the day.

After-School Programs Make A Difference

After-school programs, whether run by schools, churches, or other community groups, provide positive environments and enriching activities that truly interest and benefit teens. For some teenagers, they can make the difference between failure and success as they get ready to enter the adult world.

In after-school programs, teens can participate in a variety of interesting and challenging activities. Some programs give teens a chance to learn to play an instrument, learn a new sport, or join a theatre troupe. In others, teens learn to work with computers, get help with homework, or make a difference by volunteering in their communities.

Quality after-school programs have been shown to do the following:

- decrease juvenile crime

- decrease the likelihood that teens will be victims of violent crime

- decrease teen participation in risky behaviors, such as drug, alcohol, and tobacco use

- lead teens to develop new skills and interests

- improve teens' grades and academic achievement

- encourage teens to reach higher in planning their futures

- increase teens' self-confidence and social skills

What You Can Do

Find An After-School Program That Is Right For You

After-school programs give you a great chance to meet new people, explore new interests, and develop new talents and skills. Here are some ways you can find a program that is right for you:

- **Check with your school.** Ask a teacher or the principal at your school about whether your school offers an after-school program.

- **A number of other organizations in your community are likely to offer after-school programs.** Depending on your interests, you may want to check with your local Parks and Recreation Department, nearby churches, synagogues, mosques, and other religious organizations, or the Police Athletic League. Check your local Yellow Pages under "Youth Organizations," "Youth Centers," or "Teen-Age Activities." Alternatively, contact the national offices of youth agencies to find their local organizations. Some national organizations that are likely to be active in your community include the YMCA, Boys and Girls Clubs of America, Girls, Inc., Camp Fire Boys and Girls, and 4-H Council.

✤ **It's A Fact!!**
After-school programs give teens the opportunity to build on what they have learned during the regular school day, explore new interests, and develop relationships with caring adults.

- **Talk to your friends and other students about what they do after school.** They may be able to tell you about good programs in your area.

Encourage Your Friends And Others To Participate In After-School Programs

- Learn as much as you can about local after-school programs. If necessary, recruit an adult to help you make telephone calls for more information.

- Ask your teachers to learn about their students' work in after-school programs and highlight their work and accomplishments during class when it relates to the class or lesson subject.

♣ It's A Fact!!
Too Few Teens Have Access To Quality After-School Programs

Not enough after-school programs are available for teens. In one recent survey the following was found to be true:

- More than half of the teens (52 percent) said they wished more after-school activities were available in their neighborhood or community.

- Six in ten teens (62 percent) that were currently unsupervised during the week said they would be likely to participate in after-school programs if they were available.

- More than one-half of the teens (54 percent) said they would watch less television or play fewer video games if they had other things to do after school.

- Encourage other students to share their work in after-school programs during the school day. Publicize their work in the school newspaper, the yearbook, on bulletin boards, displays in the school library and elsewhere, and morning announcements. Ask appropriate teachers and student staff to devote a regular portion of the school newsletter and school bulletin boards to news of local after-school programs.

- Ask your teachers and school administration to offer space to after-school programs for performances, art shows, sports, and other activities.

Support The Development Of Quality After-School Programs In Your Community

These are a few steps you can take to generate interest and gain the support of adults who can help make an after-school program happen:

1. Drum up interest in starting an after-school program in your community by talking to friends, parents, guardians, and neighbors.

2. List everyone interested in having an after-school program. This will show just how great a desire there is in your community for such a program. Place bulletins in your school newspaper, in the PTA publication,

and around school, and make an announcement over the intercom at school to see how many others are willing to help you organize an after-school program.

3. Talk with your school principal and other school staff and teachers. Principals often decide who can use school facilities and equipment after school. Your principal and teachers can be a huge help in getting people together to start an after-school program, and ask them for ideas and help in starting a program.

4. Contact others in your community who might be willing to lend a hand. For example, make calls to local political officials and the school board; the neighborhood police; the mayor and city council members; local YMCAs; the parks and recreation director; local business leaders; Boys & Girls Clubs; 4-H staff; community centers; libraries; and local churches, synagogues, mosques, and other religious centers, to round up support and enthusiasm. Ask them to commit their energy and ideas, time, and even money to help start an after-school program in your community.

5. Help organize a meeting for everyone who wants to help start an after-school program. At the meeting, talk about the benefits of having a meaningful program to the community. Assign people at the meeting to complete various tasks that will eventually lead to the creation of an after-school program. Some of the tasks you will assign include finding out how other communities started after-school programs, developing a fundraising plan, and determining what you need to create an after-school program.

6. Encourage everyone involved to give serious thought to the design of the after-school program. Read about the different types of after-school programs that have been shown to be effective in making a difference in the lives of children and teens, and learn about the key elements of quality programs. The report, *Working for Children and Families: Safe and Smart After-School Programs* (http://www.ed.gov), is a good place to start.

7. Participate regularly. Once an after-school program is a reality, make sure you, and all those who played a key role in getting it off the ground, become regular participants.

Chapter 42

Conflict Resolution

Getting Along With Others

Someone took your seat at lunch or pushed ahead of you in line. Your best friend wants you to let her cheat off your test paper. A guy in math class called you something not so nice. Sometimes it seems like life is a sea of problems, and your ship is sinking.

In every situation, everyone sees things differently and wants to do things their way. It is normal for people to believe they are right, which leads to disagreements. Problems are never fun; but they can help you to have a good discussion, and you can work things out. Clearing the air will help you learn more about your friends, your family, and even yourself. Solving problems in the right way can also help you get through them quickly and easily, and stop them from getting out of control, or even violent.

About This Chapter: Information under the heading "Getting Along With Others" is from "BAM! Guide to Getting Along," BAM! Body and Mind, Centers for Disease Control and Prevention, 2003. Text under the heading "Mediation" is from "What Is Mediation?" *Youth in action*, Number 15, March 2000, Office of Juvenile Justice and Delinquency Prevention, Office of Justice Programs, U.S. Department of Justice; http://www.ncjrs.gov/html/ojjdp/youthbulletin/2000_03_1/1.html; accessed January 2007. Despite the older date of this document, the information presented is still appropriate for readers seeking to understand mediation.

If sparks do start to fly, you have the power to put out the fire. The next time you have an issue on your hands, do not explode or let someone walk all over you. Instead, convince them to try working things out with you.

Iron Out Your Issues

No plan will magically solve every problem or situation, but here are some ideas that have worked like a charm for other people:

- **Take a moment.** Stepping back from the whole mess gives everyone a chance to cool down and think. When you are having a problem with someone, first take some time to understand your own thoughts and feelings. What is really the issue? For example, do you feel like you are not getting enough respect? What do you want? Why? Next, find a time to work out the problem with the other person. Pick a quiet place where it is easy to talk. Make sure to give yourself enough time. (Out by the school buses 15 minutes before soccer practice probably is not a good choice.)

> ✔ **Quick Tip**
> **Put It On Simmer**
>
> Feel like you are about to lose it? Here are some tips to keep your anger from boiling over:
>
> 1. Take some deep breaths and concentrate on relaxing your body with each breath.
>
> 2. Count to ten slowly.
>
> 3. Think before you react. What are the consequences of your actions?
>
> 4. Keep your voice low and slow.
>
> 5. Split the scene. Remove yourself from the situation. Leave the room for a minute or take a short walk.
>
> Source: Centers for Disease Control and Prevention, 2003.

- **Set the tone.** The "tone" is the mood of the talk. When you wake up in a bad mood, it can spoil the whole day. You want to make sure that your talk at least starts off with a good mood. Just saying, "Let's work this out" can make a huge difference.

- **Agree on the problem.** Take turns telling your sides of the story. You cannot solve a problem if you do not really understand everything that is going on.

When it is your turn, see how calm you can be. Speak softly, slowly, and firmly. No threats (like "If you don't shut up, I'll..."), because they can raise the problem to a whole new level—a bad one. No need to get all excited or mad.

Try giving your point of view this way: "I feel ____(angry, sad, or upset) when you____ (take my stuff without permission, call me a name, or leave me out) because___ (you should ask first, it hurts my feelings, or makes me feel lonely)." This really works to get people to listen because they do not feel like you are judging them. Check out the difference. You could say "You're always late to pick me up!" or "I feel embarrassed when you pick me up late because all of my friends leave right on time, and it seems like no one remembered me." You can also try just stating the facts. Instead of saying "You're a thief!" try "Maybe you picked up my shirt by mistake."

When it is the other person's turn, let them explain. Listen. Do not interrupt. Try to understand where they are coming from. Show that you hear them. When people are not getting along, each person is part of the problem, but most of us tend to blame the other person. When you have done something wrong, be ready to say you are sorry.

The goal is to decide together what the real issues are. Do not pass "Go" until you do that.

✔ Quick Tip
When Is A Conflict Not A Conflict At All?

When you stop it before it starts. Lots of times, problems start when someone does not understand where another person is coming from. (Remember the last time someone got mad at you for what seemed like no reason?) So, if you are confused about why someone is acting weird or mean, find out why. Talk, e-mail, IM, send a text message. When they tell you, really listen. If someone tries to make you mad on purpose, just ignore them or ask them why. No one controls your feelings but you.

Source: Centers for Disease Control and Prevention, 2003.

Think Of Solutions

Take turns coming up with ways to solve the problem. Get creative. Usually, there are lots of possible solutions. Next, talk about the good and bad points of each one.

Make A Deal

Then, choose a solution that you both can agree on. Pick an idea that you both think will work. Get into the specifics, and talk about exactly who will do what and when you will do it. Everyone should give something.

> ✔ **Quick Tip**
> **Can't Solve It?**
>
> Sometimes that is okay. Just agree to disagree. You can still get along even if you do not see eye-to-eye on a certain thing.
>
> Source: Centers for Disease Control and Prevention, 2003.

Stick Like Glue

Keep your word and stick to what you agreed to. Give your compromise a chance. See if it sent your problem up in smoke or if the fires are still burning.

Know When To Get Help

Sometimes a problem gets really serious. If you are not talking, and you do not trust each other, you might need another person to step in. If it looks like the problem might turn into a fight, it is definitely time to get help. Someone like a teacher, parent, or religious advisor can help calm things down so you can safely talk out the problem with the other person.

Cool Rules

Ever notice how quickly people get angry? It seems like people can go from totally happy to totally ticked off in no time at all. In fact, the feeling of anger is actually a series of reactions that happen in just 1/30th of a second.

The amazing thing about anger is that it is not a basic emotion like happiness. It is actually a secondary emotion, and it is supposed to help keep you safe and protect you from danger—the old fight or flight thing; but if it gets out of hand, or if you try to ignore it, it can lead to some serious issues. Here is how to break the chain:

- **Stop it at the first spark.** Lots of things can trigger anger, like losing a soccer game, having to deal with your bossy little sister, or your computer crashing when you are in the middle of IM'ing your pals or writing a school paper. The important thing is to figure out what is really making you angry. Is it the same thing every time or do different things bring you to the boiling point? If it is always the same situation, person, or thing, try to avoid it. If you cannot avoid them (because you know your little sister is not going anywhere), think of different ways you can keep from getting angry. Instead of hurling the computer out the window, think about how you avoid it crashing to begin with, like not having your e-mail and a game going at the same time. If losing the soccer game has got your goat, use your anger as motivation to improve your skills.

- **What's it all mean?** So, snaps for figuring out how to spot the things you know make you angry, but your little sister is still driving you nuts. Since she is staying put, you have got to figure out a way to handle your anger that will not make things worse. This brings us to the second link in the chain. To avoid it, all you need to do is try to look at things from her point of view—you are older, and she wants to hang with you because she thinks you are cool. With that in mind, it is easier to keep your cool. Spend some time just with her so that she will not need to stalk you when all your friends are over. You might even find out that she is not half bad. By changing the way you deal with her and understanding her point of view, you can break the anger chain before you even notice you are mad.

- **Blood's a boiling.** Well, okay, but you are still furious. You have tried to change your reactions to the things that you know make you crazy, you are busy looking at everything from everyone else's point of view, but you can still feel your temperature is rising. That is your body responding to your feelings. You get hot, and your muscles might start to tighten, and you start breathing harder. Do not let it get the best of you. There are things you can do to stay in control. Take some deep breaths, focus on relaxing your muscles, and slow down.

- **Talking to yourself?** The next link in the chain comes when you catch yourself thinking or saying something in reaction to what is happening to make you mad. We have all done it. We think things like "He's so stupid" or say to a friend "You're always so mean!" before we can stop ourselves. If you catch yourself doing this, take a minute to think. Try to remember that you are dealing with a person who may not know how you feel. Stay calm. Lashing back will not get you anywhere, so try to talk to your friend, let him know he hurt your feelings, and then try to move on.

- **What you've got to do with it.** The way you feel in a situation depends on your background. You may be used to people keeping their feelings in and not talking about them, or you may be used to people exploding and yelling when they are angry. Neither of these reactions is necessarily good. People who bottle up their feelings can end up exploding later or becoming depressed. People who vent and yell just tend to keep the anger cycle in motion. The trick is to deal with your anger so

---

✔ Quick Tip

- Figure out what methods work for you to control your anger.

- Talk to an adult you trust if you feel intensely angry, fearful, or anxious.

- Do not carry weapons or associate with people who do. Weapons escalate conflicts and increase the chances of serious harm. It is also illegal for a teen to carry a handgun; you can be arrested and charged with a crime.

- Avoid or be cautious in places or situations where conflicts tend to arise such as crowded hallways, bathrooms, or unsupervised places in a school.

- Reject taunts for a fight and find a compromise to a dispute rather than resorting to violence.

- Decide on your options for handling a problem when conflict arises such as talking the problem out calmly, staying away from certain people, or getting others involved to settle a dispute such as a teacher, peer mediator, or counselor.

- Understand that retaliation (getting back at someone in a violent way) is not an effective way to respond to teasing, insults, rough play, and offensive touching (pushing, grabbing, shoving, slapping, kicking or hitting).

Source: Excerpted from "Conflict Resolution," National Youth Violence Prevention Resource Center, October 2005.

that you can learn how to not get riled up in the first place. Try these suggestions to stay cool, calm, and collected:

- Go for a walk.

- Write down your feelings on a piece of paper, then tear it up and throw it away.

- Face the mirror and practice talking to the person that you are mad at.

- **That's the way the story ends.** Isn't it amazing how many things come in between the first spark and being really mad? The whole chain happens so fast because we train ourselves to react in a certain way without even knowing we are doing it; but if you learn to recognize the steps in between, you can break the chain before you lose your cool. No matter how hard you try, you will not be able to avoid getting angry in every situation. You just have to decide the best way to respond. Anger does not have to be negative. If you handle it the right way, it can actually clue you in to dangerous situations and make you a stronger person.

Mediation

What Is Mediation?

In a process called mediation, a person trained as a mediator helps two (or more) people resolve a conflict or disagreement. The conflict being resolved might be as simple as who should pay for a damaged locker, or it might be as complex as which parent should receive custody of a child in the case of a divorce. In either situation, mediation involves solving the dispute through peaceful means. The mediator, however, does not simply listen to the conflict and draw up the terms of a solution; the people with the conflict (the participants or disputants) do that. In addition, it is the participants, not the mediator, who enforce the agreed-upon solution.

The mediator plays a special role. He or she does not decide what is right or wrong or find people guilty or innocent, as a judge would in a courtroom. Instead, the mediator tries to help the disputants find, and agree upon, a peaceful way to resolve their conflict.

How Does Mediation Prevent Or Reduce Crime?

As you know, conflict is an unavoidable part of life. Passengers in a car might disagree about a wrong turn on a road trip. A person may play music more loudly than others would like. Friends may argue over who is to blame for a broken possession. These are all types of conflict.

Conflicts are not always minor and harmless. Assaults or threatened assaults often happen between people who know each other and, in many of these cases, start off with small arguments or disagreements. The mediation process provides a way for these people to resolve their disagreements before either party resorts to violence. It also helps people reach agreements without feeling they have had to "give in." In this way, both sides in mediation come out winners.

Mediation has helped to reduce violence in neighborhoods and in schools. Using peers as mediators—a process known as "peer mediation"—is a popular way of handling conflicts and preventing violence in middle schools and high schools. Schools using this process recruit and train students interested in being peer mediators. Guidance counselors, or other trained professionals, teach the young mediators how to listen to both sides of an argument, offer unbiased impressions, and help students in conflict find a workable solution to their problem.

Peer mediators help the disputants re-channel anger and reach peaceful agreements. When a disagreement or conflict arises, a teacher, an administrator, a concerned student, or the fighting students themselves can refer the issue to peer mediation. A peer mediator is quickly assigned, and the mediation process begins, resolving the issue and preventing further discord. Playground mediators in elementary schools similarly help prevent fights and resolve disagreements between much younger students.

Sample Mediation Session

Step 1: Introduction

The mediator's first job is to make the parties feel at ease and explain the ground rules. The mediator's role is not to make a decision but to help the parties reach agreement. The mediator explains that he or she will not take sides.

Step 2: Telling The Story

Each party tells what happened. One person tells his or her side of the story first. No interruptions are allowed. The other party then explains his or her version of the facts. Again, no interruptions are allowed. Any of the participants, including the mediator, may take notes during the process. The mediator's notes are thrown away at the end of the session to ensure confidentiality.

Step 3: Identifying Facts, Issues, And Interests

The mediator next attempts to identify any agreed-upon facts and issues and the issues that are important to each person. The mediator listens to each side, summarizes each party's view, and checks to make sure each party understands the other's view.

Step 4: Identifying Alternative Solutions

During this step, the participants (with help from the mediator) think of all possible solutions to their problem. Because the opposing sides to the dispute probably arrived at the mediation session with a desired outcome in mind, it is often difficult for them to consider other solutions. The mediator makes a list of solutions and asks each party to explain his or her feelings about each one.

Step 5: Revising And Discussing Solutions

On the basis of feelings expressed by each party, the mediator revises the list of possible solutions and tries to identify a solution that both parties may be able to agree on.

Step 6: Reaching An Agreement

The mediator helps the parties to reach an agreement by choosing a solution that has been discussed and that both parties agree on. After the parties have decided on a solution, an agreement should be put in writing. The written agreement should be as specific as possible, stating exactly what each party has agreed to do and when he or she will do it. The agreement should also explain what will happen if either disputant breaks the agreement. Some agreements require parties to appear for additional mediation; others call for the payment of money or the performance of services when an agreement is broken. In most instances, the parties themselves are responsible for enforcing the contract by bringing examples of breached agreements to the attention of the mediation program. Once it is finalized, both parties sign the agreement, which usually takes the form of a contract, is signed by both parties.

Chapter 43

Is Your Relationship A Healthy One?

Sometimes it feels impossible to find someone who's right for you—and who thinks you're right for him or her. So when it happens, you're usually so psyched that you don't even mind when your little brother finishes all the ice cream or your English teacher chooses the one day when you didn't do your reading to give you a pop quiz.

It's totally normal to look at the world through rose-colored glasses in the early stages of a relationship. But for some people, those rose-colored glasses turn into blinders that keep them from seeing that a relationship isn't as healthy as it should be.

What Makes A Healthy Relationship?

Hopefully, you and your significant other are treating each other fabulously. Not sure if that's the case? Take a step back from the dizzying sensation of being swept off your feet and think about whether your relationship has these qualities:

- **Mutual Respect:** Does he or she get how cool you are and why? (Watch out if the answer to the first part is yes but only because you're acting

About This Chapter: Information in this chapter is from "Am I in a Healthy Relationship?" This information was provided by TeensHealth, one of the largest resources online for medically reviewed health information written for teens, kids, and parents. For more articles like this one, visit www.TeensHealth.org, or www.KidsHealth.org. © 2005 The Nemours Foundation.

like someone you're not.) The key is that your boyfriend or girlfriend is into you for who you are—for your great sense of humor, your love of reality TV, etc. Does your partner listen when you say you're not comfortable doing something and then back off right away? Respect in a relationship means that each person values whom the other is and understands—and would never challenge—the other person's boundaries.

- **Trust:** You're talking with a guy from French class, and your boyfriend walks by. Does he completely lose his cool or keep walking because he knows you'd never cheat on him? It's OK to get a little jealous sometimes—jealousy is a natural emotion. But how a person reacts when he or she feels jealous is what matters. There's no way you can have a healthy relationship if you don't trust each other.

- **Honesty:** This one goes hand-in-hand with trust, because it's tough to trust someone when one of you isn't being honest. Have you ever caught your girlfriend in a major lie? Like she told you that she had to work on Friday night, but it turned out she was at the movies with her friends? The next time she says she has to work, you'll have a lot more trouble believing her, and the trust will be on shaky ground.

- **Support:** It's not just in bad times that your partner should support you. Some people are great when your whole world is falling apart but can't take being there when things are going right (and vice versa). In a healthy relationship, your significant other is there with a shoulder to cry on when you find out your parents are getting divorced and to celebrate with you when you get the lead in a play.

- **Fairness/Equality:** You need to have give-and-take in your relationship, too. Do you take turns choosing which new movie to see? As a couple, do you hang out with your partner's friends as often as you hang out with yours? It's not like you have to keep a running count and make sure things are exactly even, of course. But you'll know if it isn't a pretty fair balance. Things get bad really fast when a relationship turns into a power struggle, with one person fighting to get his or her way all the time.

- **Separate Identities:** In a healthy relationship, everyone needs to make compromises. But that doesn't mean you should feel like you're losing out on being yourself. When you started going out, you both had your own lives—your own families, friends, interests, hobbies, etc.—and that shouldn't change. Neither of you should have to pretend to like something you don't, or give up seeing your friends, or drop out of activities you love. And you also should feel free to keep developing new talents or interests, making new friends, and moving forward.

- **Good Communication:** You've probably heard lots of stuff about how men and women don't seem to speak the same language. We all know how many different meanings the little phrase "no, nothing's wrong" can have, depending on who's saying it. But what's important is to ask if you're not sure what he or she means, and speak honestly and openly so that the miscommunication is avoided in the first place. Never keep a feeling bottled up because you're afraid it's not what your boyfriend or girlfriend wants to hear or because you worry about sounding silly. And if you need some time to think something through before you're ready to talk about it, the right person will give you some space to do that if you ask for it.

What's An Unhealthy Relationship?

Some people live in homes with parents who fight a lot or abuse each other—emotionally or physically. For some people who have grown up around this kind of behavior it can almost seem normal or OK. It's not. Many of us learn from watching and imitating the people close to us. So someone who has lived around violent or disrespectful behavior may not have learned how to treat others with kindness and respect or how to expect the same treatment.

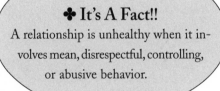

✤ It's A Fact!!
A relationship is unhealthy when it involves mean, disrespectful, controlling, or abusive behavior.

Qualities like kindness and respect are absolute requirements for a healthy relationship. Someone who doesn't yet have this part down may need to work on it with a trained therapist before he or she is ready for a relationship. Meanwhile, even though you may feel bad or feel for someone who's been mistreated, you need to take care of yourself—it's not healthy to stay in a relationship that involves abusive behavior of any kind.

Warning Signs

Here's some scary news: In one survey, 20% of American girls reported having been hit, slapped, or forced into sexual activity by their partners. This stuff happens to guys, too—they are just less likely to report it. And 40% of all teens said they know someone at school who experienced dating violence. So if you think there's no way it could happen to you or someone you know, think again.

Ask yourself, does my boyfriend or girlfriend do the following:

- get angry when I don't drop everything for him or her?

- criticize the way I look or dress, and say I'll never be able to find anyone else who would date me?

☞ Remember!!
No one deserves to be hit, shoved, or forced into anything he or she doesn't want to do.

- keep me from seeing friends or from talking to any other guys or girls?

- want me to quit an activity, even though I love it?

- ever raise a hand when angry, like he or she is about to hit me?

- try to force me to go further sexually than I want to?

These aren't the only questions you can ask yourself. If you can think of any way in which your boyfriend or girlfriend is trying to control you, make you feel bad about yourself, isolate you from the rest of your world, or—this is a big one—harm you physically or sexually, then it's time to get out, fast. Let a trusted friend or family member know what's going on and make sure you're safe. It can be tempting to make excuses or misinterpret violence as an expression of love. But even if you know that the person hurting you loves you, it is not healthy.

Why Are Some Relationships So Difficult?

Ever heard about how it's hard for someone to love you when you don't love yourself? It's a big relationship roadblock when one or both people struggle with self-esteem problems. Your girlfriend or boyfriend isn't there to make you feel good about yourself if you can't do that on your own. Focus on being happy with yourself, and don't take on the responsibility of worrying about someone else's happiness.

What if you feel that your girlfriend or boyfriend needs too much from you? If the relationship feels like a burden or a drag instead of a joy, it may be time to think about whether it's a healthy match for you. Someone who's not happy or secure may have trouble being a healthy relationship partner.

Also, intense relationships can be hard for some teenagers. Some are so focused on their own developing feelings and responsibilities that they don't have the emotional energy it takes to respond to someone else's feelings and needs in a close relationship. Don't worry if you're just not ready yet. You will be, and you can take all the time you need.

Ever notice that some teen relationships don't last very long? It's no wonder—you're still growing and changing every day, and it can be tough to put two people together whose identities are both still in the process of forming. You two might seem perfect for each other at first, but that can change. If you try to hold on to the relationship anyway, there's a good chance it will turn sour. Better to part as friends than to stay in something that you've outgrown or that no longer feels right for one or both of you. And before you go looking for amour from that hottie from French class, respect your current beau by breaking things off before you make your move.

Relationships can be one of the best—and most challenging—parts of your world. They can be full of fun, romance, excitement, intense feelings, and occasional heartache, too. Whether you're single or in a relationship, remember that it's good to be choosy about who you get close to. If you're still waiting, take your time and get to know plenty of people. Think about the qualities you value in a friendship and see how they match up with the ingredients of a healthy relationship. Work on developing those good qualities in yourself—they make you a lot more attractive to others. And if you're already part of a pair, make sure the relationship you're in brings out the best in both of you.

Chapter 44

How To Help A Friend Who Is Abused At Home

Here's how you can help a friend who is being abused or who is living in a family where there is abuse or domestic violence.

Keep in mind that supporting someone who's living with abuse is difficult. Remember that even people with lots of power, like the police and courts, can find it hard to protect people from abuse, so this is not a situation that you can "fix" on your own. You may need to talk to an adult.

What To Say To A Friend

- **Tell them you are worried about them and ask if they are okay.** For example, say, "I've noticed you seem really down lately. Is everything okay?"

- **Let them know that you believe them** by telling them that or saying something like "I'm glad that you told me."

  "When Anna first told me I was like, what? Your family? I always thought that her family was the coolest. First off I almost went 'no way', but then I

About This Chapter: Information in this chapter is from "Knowing Your Friends Business." Adapted with permission from www.burstingthebubble.com, an educational website developed by the Domestic Violence and Incest Resource Centre, Victoria, Australia, © 2003. All rights reserved.

saw the look on her face, so I just went, 'Anna, that's horrible. I had no idea.'"

- **Reassure them that the abuse is not their fault** by saying, "No one deserves to be treated like that" or "I think that what is happening is so wrong!"

"When Dale started staying away from school and coming in with bruises and stuff, I said to him one day, 'This is crap, man. No one should have to put up with that crap.'"

- **Don't push them to tell you details** about what's happened unless they really want to. Some people may be dying to talk about it, while others may feel upset by having to re-tell the details. Also, you may find it too full on to deal with.

- **Let them know that this happens to other people, too.** Other young people have dealt with this in their families—they are not alone.

- **Let them know there are people who can help.** Encourage them to tell an adult or someone else who can help. If they aren't ready for this, let them know that there are anonymous help lines that they can talk to. You could even offer to call a support service and get information for them, or you could offer to go with them to talk to an adult or a service.

> ☞ **Remember!!**
>
> Don't gossip with other friends about what your friend has told you, unless you think they can help. Getting help from an adult or someone else who can help is a good idea, though, and isn't gossiping.

"I was so mad to think that my girlfriend has to go through all that. I'd always thought that her mom's boyfriend was a pig, and when I found out what he'd done, I wanted to smash him! My girlfriend got upset and said, 'You'll just make it worse'. Eventually she decided to go to the cops, but chickened out at the last second, so asked me to call them for her."

- **Get help for yourself too.** Helping someone in this situation can be stressful for you, too. Talk to an adult that you trust, like a parent or friend's parent, or a teacher, or even a support service. You don't have to tell them which friend you were helping.

What If My Friend Won't Get Help?

If your friend doesn't want to tell anyone or get any help, it can be really hard for you, especially if you're worried about what might happen. Maybe you want to be a good friend, and you want to look out for them; but you don't want to break their trust, so what can you do?

Here's one story about what someone did when her boyfriend wanted to keep it a secret.

"My boyfriend was in a really bad situation at home, and we'd talked about it heaps. He hadn't told me all the details, but he was always really down about it. He hardly ever invited people over to his house, including me. Once I turned up there as a surprise, and he hurried me to go out instead. I could tell something was seriously wrong."

"I asked him about it, and he told me that his dad is always getting angry, and that he has bashed his mom a few times. He hit my boyfriend once, too, when he tried to stop his dad. I suggested telling a teacher or the school counselor, but he said no, he didn't want to get anyone in trouble, and he was worried he'd get taken away from home. It was hard because I was worried, but he trusted me, and anyway, I could understand him being afraid of what would happen. He just wanted his dad to treat his mother and sisters better."

"One night I called him at home, and his voice sounded really strange, really different. I heard his dad yelling, and my boyfriend said he had to get off the phone. I got worried that he could be hurt, too. The next day I told him how I felt and said I was going to ask my mom what she thought, without telling her whom it was about. He said that was okay. Well, it all came out when I spoke to my mom because I got upset, and she guessed it was my boyfriend. But actually she was so good; she invited him over, and said to him that if there's ever trouble at home, he and his sister can come over to our place. At first he didn't want to admit it, but then he ended up talking to my mom about his family, and we talked about what else he can do, like calling the

police. My mom offered to speak to his mom to see if she needs some help, and he said he would think about it."

"Now I think he's glad that he has spoken to someone about it, and we can try to help him deal with it."

Chapter 45

What Happens When Possible Abuse Or Neglect Is Reported?

How does the child welfare system work?

The child welfare system is a group of services designed to promote the well-being of children by ensuring safety, achieving permanency, and strengthening families to successfully care for their children. Most families first become involved with the child welfare system due to a report of suspected child abuse or neglect (sometimes called "child maltreatment"). Federal law defines child maltreatment as serious harm (neglect, physical abuse, sexual abuse, and emotional abuse or neglect) caused to children by parents or primary caregivers such as extended family members or babysitters. Child maltreatment also can include harm that a caregiver allows to happen, or does not prevent from happening, to a child. In general, child welfare agencies do not intervene in cases of harm to children caused by acquaintances or strangers. These cases are the responsibility of law enforcement.

The child welfare system is not a single entity. Many organizations in each community work together to strengthen families and keep children safe. Public agencies, such as departments of social services or child and family

About This Chapter: Information in this chapter is from "How Does the Child Welfare System Work?" Child Welfare Information Gateway (www.childwelfare.gov), Children's Bureau, Administration for Children, Youth and Families, U.S. Department of Health and Human Services, December 2006.

services, often contract and collaborate with private child welfare agencies and community-based organizations to provide services to families such as in-home family preservation services, foster care, residential treatment, mental health care, substance abuse treatment, parenting skills classes, employment assistance, and financial or housing assistance.

Child welfare systems are complex, and their specific procedures vary widely by state. The purpose of this chapter is to give a brief overview of the purposes and functions of child welfare from a national perspective. Child welfare systems typically do the following:

- receive and investigate reports of possible child abuse and neglect

- provide services to families who need assistance in the protection and care of their children

- arrange for children to live with foster families when they are not safe at home

- arrange permanent adoptive homes or independent living services for children leaving foster care

What happens when possible abuse or neglect is reported?

Any concerned person can report suspicions of child abuse or neglect. Most reports are made by people who are required by state law to report suspicions of child abuse and neglect—mandatory reporters. In approximately 18 states and Puerto Rico, any person who suspects child abuse or neglect is required to report. Reports of possible child abuse and neglect are generally received by child protective services (CPS) workers and either "screened in" or "screened out." A report is screened in if there is sufficient information to suggest an investigation is warranted. A report may be screened out if there is not enough information on which to follow up or if the situation reported does not meet the state's legal definition of abuse or neglect. In these instances, the worker may refer the person reporting the incident to other community services or law enforcement for additional help.

What happens after a report is screened in?

CPS workers, often called investigators, respond within a particular time period, which may be anywhere from a few hours to a few days, depending on the type of maltreatment alleged, the potential severity of the situation, and requirements under state law. They may speak with the parents and other people in contact with the child such as doctors, teachers, or childcare providers. They also may speak with the child, alone or in the presence of caregivers, depending on the child's age and level of risk. Children who are believed to be in immediate danger may be moved to a shelter, foster care placement, or a relative's home during the investigation and while court proceedings are pending. An investigator's primary purpose is to determine if abuse or neglect has occurred and if there is a risk of it occurring again.

Some jurisdictions now employ an alternative response system. In these jurisdictions, when risk to the children involved is considered to be low, the CPS caseworker may focus on assessing family difficulties and offering needed services, rather than gathering evidence to confirm the occurrence of abuse or neglect.

At the end of an investigation, CPS workers typically make one of two findings—"unsubstantiated" ("unfounded") or "substantiated" ("founded"). These terms vary from state to state. Typically, a finding of "unsubstantiated" means there is insufficient evidence for the worker to conclude that a child was abused or neglected, or what happened does not meet the legal definition of child abuse or neglect. A finding of "substantiated" typically means an incident of child abuse or neglect, as defined by state law, is believed to have occurred. Some states have additional categories, such as "unable to determine," that suggest there was not enough evidence to either confirm or refute that abuse or neglect occurred.

The agency will initiate a court action if it determines that the authority of the juvenile court (through a child protection or dependency proceeding) is necessary to keep the child safe. To protect the child, the court can issue temporary orders placing the child in shelter care during the investigation, ordering services, or ordering certain individuals to have no contact with the child. At an adjudicatory hearing, the court hears evidence and decides whether maltreatment occurred and whether the child should be under the continuing jurisdiction of the court. The court then enters a disposition, either at that hearing or at a separate hearing, which may result in the court ordering a parent to comply with services necessary to ameliorate the abuse or neglect. Orders can also contain provisions regarding visitation between the parent and the child, agency obligations to provide the parent with services, and services needed by the child.

♣ It's A Fact!!

In 2004, approximately 872,000 children were found to be victims of child abuse or neglect.

What happens in substantiated cases?

If a child has been abused or neglected, the course of action depends on state policy, the severity of the maltreatment, the risk of continued or future maltreatment, the services available to address the family's needs, and whether the child was removed from the home and a court action to protect the child was initiated. The following general options are available:

- **No Or Low Risk:** The family's case may be closed with no services if the maltreatment was a one-time incident, there is no or low risk of future incidents, or the services the family needs will not be provided through the child welfare agency but through other systems.

- **Low To Moderate Risk:** Referrals may be made to community-based or voluntary in-home CPS services if the CPS worker believes the family would benefit from these services and the risk to the child would be lessened. This may happen even when no abuse or neglect is found, if the family needs and is willing to participate in the services.

- **Moderate To High Risk:** The family may again be offered voluntary in-home CPS services to help ameliorate the risks. If these are refused, the agency may seek intervention by the juvenile dependency court. Once there is a judicial determination that abuse or neglect occurred, juvenile dependency court may require the family to cooperate with in-home CPS services if it is believed that the child can remain safely at home while the family addresses the issues contributing to the risk of future maltreatment. If the child has been seriously harmed or is considered to be at high risk of serious harm, the court may order the child's removal from the home or affirm the agency's prior removal of the child. The child may be placed with a relative or in foster care.

What happens to people who abuse children?

People who are found to have abused or neglected a child are generally offered voluntary help or required by a juvenile dependency court to participate in services that will help keep their children safe. In more severe cases or fatalities, police are called upon to investigate and may file charges in criminal court against the perpetrators of child maltreatment. In many states certain types of abuse, such as sexual abuse and serious physical abuse, are routinely referred to law enforcement.

Whether or not criminal charges are filed, the perpetrator's name may be placed on a state child maltreatment registry if abuse or neglect is confirmed. A registry is a central database that collects information about maltreated children and individuals who were found to have abused or neglected those children. These registries are usually confidential and used for internal child protective purposes only. However, they may be used in background checks for certain professions, such as those working with children, so children will be protected from contact with individuals who may mistreat them.

What happens to children who enter foster care?

Most children in foster care are placed with relatives or foster families, but some may be placed in group homes. While a child is in foster care, he or she attends school and should receive medical care and other services as needed. The child's family also receives services to support their efforts to reduce the risk of future maltreatment and to help them, in most cases, to be reunited with their child. Parents may visit their children on a predetermined basis. Visits also are arranged between siblings, if they cannot be placed together.

Every child in foster care should have a permanency plan that

♣ **It's A Fact!!**

In 2004, an estimated 268,000 children were removed from their homes as a result of a child abuse investigation or assessment.

describes where the child will live after he or she leaves foster care. Families typically participate in developing a permanency plan for the child and a service plan for the family. These plans guide the agency's work. Except in unusual and extreme circumstances, every child's plan is first focused on re-unification with parents. If the efforts toward reunification are not successful, the plan may be changed to another permanent arrangement such as adoption or transfer of custody to a relative. Occasionally, the plan involves a permanent placement with a foster family, usually for older children who have become strongly attached to the family or for whom a suitable adoptive home cannot be found. In addition to a permanency plan, older children should receive transitional or independent living services to assist them in being self-sufficient when they leave foster care between the ages of 18 and 21.

Federal law requires the court to hold a permanency hearing, which determines the permanent plan for the child, within 12 months after the child enters foster care and every 12 months thereafter. Many courts review each case more frequently to ensure that the agency is actively engaged in permanency planning for the child.

Chapter 46

Creating A Safety Plan

A Teen's Safety Plan

If you are in an abusive situation and are not able or ready to leave it, it is important to think about how to keep yourself safe. If you do want to leave, it is a good idea to plan your escape well. Creating a safety plan can help you feel safe whether you are staying in your current situation or getting ready to leave. Be sure to review it every so often with someone you trust to keep the information useful and up-to-date. Use the form shown in Figure 46.1 to create your safety plan.

Tips For Safety And Confidence

- Stand up for yourself. If the abuse is just starting, tell the abuser that his/her behavior is not acceptable and that you will not put up with it. Talk to a trusted adult or peer about what is happening.

- Be careful. If the abuse is ongoing and the abuser is accustomed to getting his/her own way, you may risk more violence if you stand up for yourself. If you are afraid this might happen, try to get support from an adult or friend before you make a stand. Do not try it when you are alone with the abuser, and be prepared to take the step of leaving in order to escape the abuse.

About This Chapter: Information in this chapter is reprinted with permission from the Family Violence Prevention Fund, www.endabuse.org. Copyright © 2007 Family Violence Prevention Fund. All rights reserved.

Figure 46.1. A Teen's Safety Plan

I will tell (name): _____ and
(name): _____ about the abuse and ask
them to help me if I use the code word or phrase:

_____

or if they learn I am being hurt by any other means.

I will buy a small address book and carry it with me at all times. I will list the following people, agencies, shelters, hotlines, or other services in the book:

1. _____

2. _____

3. _____

I will make a habit of leaving as often as possible to:

_____

I will use this excuse when I am able or ready to leave the situation.

I will leave before I think a situation will get violent. I usually know things are getting violent when:
_____

My abuser may try to persuade me not to leave by:
_____

_____

I can get around this by:
_____

_____

If I decide to leave, I will go to either of the following places that are unknown to my abuser:

1. _____

2. _____

I will keep the following items in a bag that is ready to go (those that apply):

- keys
- address book
- driver's license or other identification
- social security card
- school records
- passport
- resident card
- immigration papers
- bus tokens
- spare change
- small amount of cash
- checkbook
- spare clothes
- pager
- restraining/protection orders
- rent papers
- current unpaid bills
- insurance papers
- prescriptions/medicines
- special photos
- personal items

For teens with children, have the following ready: formula and bottle, diapers, birth certificate, child's medical records, spare clothes for child, and child's favorite toys.

If I leave, I will bring this bag, as well as:

_____

_____with me.

I will keep spare items, supplies, copies of important papers, and:

_____

with (name): _____in case I am unable to get my bag before leaving.

I will review my safety plan on (date): _____

with (name): _____

- Remember that the abuse is not your fault. Do not be ashamed to tell someone about the abuse. It is not your fault; it is the abuser's problem. Encourage him/her to get help.

- Hurting yourself is not the answer. It is normal to feel down when you are being hurt. Some people who are being abused feel like suicide is the only real option. If you feel this way, it might be because you believe the abuser's put-downs or because you are turning your anger on yourself. Use your anger instead to take care of yourself. There really are options and steps you can take to make things better for yourself. Praise yourself for what you do well and have faith in your future. If you are feeling suicidal, it may help to talk to someone about your feelings, and you can call the 24-hour Hopeline at 1-800-SUICIDE (784-2433).

- Tell someone about the abuse. Sometimes just talking about the abuse can make you feel better. At other times, an adult or friend might have useful advice or be able to offer help.

- Be careful with alcohol and drugs. Many people use alcohol and drugs to deal with tension or pain. Unfortunately, they will only drain your energy, keep you helpless, and affect your ability to think clearly.

- Relax and play. Relieving stress can improve your ability to communicate and make decisions. Physical activity can increase your sense of well-being. Regular exercise done with others can be fun, too.

- Try to eat well. Your physical health affects the way you feel as well as your ability to cope with stress.

- Save money and get some job skills. Knowing you have an emergency fund can help reduce your anxiety. If you have job skills, it will be easier to avoid depending on others to get by. Even if you cannot get a job or do not need one, you can do volunteer work to gain skills and meet new people.

- Know your local resources. To learn about domestic violence agencies in your area, call the National Domestic Violence Hotline 24 hours, 1-800-799-SAFE (7233), 1-800-787-3224 (TTY).

- Look after yourself. You are a strong person, and you can grow stronger when you know you can make it on your own. When you are ready to leave an abusive situation, know that help is there.

Chapter 47

Self-Defense

You've seen it in movies: A girl walks through an isolated parking garage. Suddenly, an evil-looking guy jumps out from behind an SUV. Girl jabs bad guy in the eyes with her keys—or maybe she kicks him in a certain sensitive place. Either way, while he's squirming, she leaps into her car and speeds to safety.

That's the movies. Here's the real-life action replay: When the girl goes to jab or kick the guy, he knows what's coming and grabs her arm (or leg), pulling her off balance. Enraged by her attempt to fight back, he flips her onto the ground. Now she's in a bad place to defend herself—and she can't run away.

Many people think of self-defense as a karate kick to the groin or jab in the eyes of an attacker. But self-defense actually means doing everything possible to avoid fighting someone who threatens or attacks you. Self-defense is all about using your smarts—not your fists.

Use Your Head

People (guys as well as girls) who are threatened and fight back "in self-defense" actually risk making a situation worse. The attacker, who is already edgy and pumped up on adrenaline—and who knows what else—may become

About This Chapter: This information was provided by TeensHealth, one of the largest resources online for medically reviewed health information written for teens, kids, and parents. For more articles like this one, visit www.TeensHealth.org, or www.KidsHealth.org. © 2006 The Nemours Foundation.

even more angry and violent. The best way to handle any attack or threat of attack is to try to get away. This way, you're least likely to be injured.

One way to avoid a potential attack before it happens is to trust your instincts. Your intuition, combined with your common sense, can help get you out of trouble. For example, if you're running alone on the school track and you suddenly feel like you're being watched, that could be your intuition telling you something. Your common sense would then tell you that it's a good idea to get back to where there are more people around.

Attackers aren't always strangers who jump out of dark alleys. Sadly, teens can be attacked by people they know. That's where another important self-defense skill comes into play. This skill is something self-defense experts and negotiators call de-escalation.

> ✔ **Quick Tip**
> **Trust Your Instincts**
> When the elevator doors open, does that shifty-looking character in the corner make you feel uneasy? Don't get on (or get off if the person who makes you uncomfortable is getting on). If you're riding the elevator and you start feeling afraid, get off on a floor where you know you'll find other people. Your safety is all about trusting your own judgment.

De-escalating a situation means speaking or acting in a way that can prevent things from getting worse. The classic example of de-escalation is giving a robber your money rather than trying to fight or run. But de-escalation can work in other ways, too. For example, if someone harasses you when there's no one else around, you can de-escalate things by agreeing with him or her. You don't have to actually believe the taunts, of course; you're just using words to get yourself out of a tight spot. Then you can redirect the bully's focus ("Oops, I just heard the bell for third period"), and calmly walk away from the situation.

Something as simple as not losing your temper can de-escalate a situation. Learn how to manage your own anger effectively so that you can talk or walk away without using your fists or weapons.

Although de-escalation won't always work, it can only help matters if you remain calm and don't give the would-be attacker any extra ammunition. Whether it's a stranger or someone you thought you could trust, saying and doing things that don't threaten your attacker can give you some control.

Reduce Your Risks

Another part of self-defense is doing things that can help you stay safe. Here are some tips from the National Crime Prevention Council and other experts:

> **✔ Quick Tip**
>
> **Fido Power:** If you have a dog, take your pooch with you when you're walking alone. Even a dog no bigger than a basket of fries can still bark or snarl enough to cause a potential attacker to think twice.

- Understand your surroundings. Walk or hang out in areas that are open, well lit, and well traveled. Become familiar with the buildings, parking lots, parks, and other places you walk. Pay particular attention to places where someone could hide—such as stairways and bushes.

- Avoid shortcuts that take you through isolated areas.

- If you're going out at night, travel in a group.

- Make sure your friends and parents know your daily schedule (classes, sports practice, club meetings, etc.). If you go on a date or with friends for an after-game snack, let someone know where you're going and when you expect to return.

- Check out hangouts. Do they look safe? Are you comfortable being there? Ask yourself if the people around you seem to share your views on fun activities—if you think they're being reckless, move on.

- Be sure your body language shows a sense of confidence. Look like you know where you're going and act alert.

- When riding on public transportation, sit near the driver and stay awake. Attackers are looking for vulnerable targets.

- Carry a cell phone if possible. Make sure it's programmed with your parents' phone number.

✔ Quick Tip: Voice Power

If you ever need help, draw attention to your situation by shouting out specific words like "Help" or "Police." Commands like "No!" or "Get away!" or "Back off!" are excellent attention-getters if you feel threatened.

- Be willing to report crimes in your neighborhood and school to the police.

Take A Self-Defense Class

The best way—in fact the only way—to prepare yourself to fight off an attacker is to take a self-defense class. We'd love to give you all the right moves in a chapter, but some things you just have to learn in person.

A good self-defense class can teach you how to size up a situation and decide what you should do. Self-defense classes can also teach special techniques for breaking an attacker's grasp and other things you can do to get away. For example, attackers usually anticipate how their victim might react—that kick to the groin or jab to the eyes, for instance. A good self-defense class can teach you ways to surprise your attacker and catch him or her off guard.

One of the best things people take away from self-defense classes is self-confidence. The last thing you want to be thinking about during an attack is, "Can I really pull this self-defense tactic off?" It's much easier to take action in an emergency if you've already had a few dry runs.

A self-defense class should give you a chance to practice your moves. If you take a class with a friend, you can continue practicing on each other to keep the moves fresh in your mind long after the class is over.

Check out your local YMCA, community hospital, or community center for classes. If they don't have them, they may be able to tell you who does. Your PE teacher or school counselor may also be a great resource.

Chapter 48

Safety On The Internet

The internet has opened up a whole new world for people of all ages. You can shop, plan a vacation, send a picture to a relative, talk with friends, and even do research for school. This new way of finding information and communicating does come with risks.

Safe Chatting

What kind of online name should I choose?

You should never use your real name as your online name. By using your real name, anyone can know right away who you are and can probably find out more about you. This is especially true in chat rooms, where you can get comfortable chatting with someone and suddenly realize they know things about you.

You probably want your online name to describe who you are, but be careful about the name and words you choose. Remember, when you are talking online to people you do not know well, some people may unfairly judge you by your online name. For example, if you choose a name like hotbabe13, people will get the wrong idea about you, and you most likely

About This Chapter: Information in this chapter is from "Safety on the Internet," "Safe chatting," and "Safe blogging," GirlsHealth.gov, sponsored by the National Women's Health Information Center, U.S. Department of Health and Human Services, August 2006.

will get unwanted e-mails from people who are just responding to your online name and not to who you really are. If you cannot think of an online name to use without describing something about yourself, try using the name of a candy bar, color, or something else that is not personal. If the name is already taken, you can try adding a few numbers, for example, Green123.

Is IMing safe?

IMing is not as private as you might think, so it is important to know how to stay safe and have fun too. Here are some tips:

- Do not respond to IMs from people you do not know or IMs that look strange. It is possible to get unwanted IMs. Like e-mails, IMs can also contain viruses.

- Do not forget to sign off when you are finished and change your password regularly. This will keep others from using your IM account.

- If you get an IM that makes you feel uncomfortable, do not respond to it. Tell your parents/guardians about it.

- Never give out your screen name or password, even to your friends.

Are chat rooms safe?

Some chat rooms are thought to be safe because the topic that is being talked about is safe, and because there is a moderator leading the chat. Even if the topic is okay, some people might talk about other things that can make you uncomfortable. If you ever feel uncomfortable or in danger for any reason, leave the chat room right away and tell a parent/guardian or other trusted adult.

☞ Remember!!

Before you enter a chat, be sure you have permission from a parent or guardian to do so.

Source: Excerpted from "Safe chatting," GirlsHealth.gov.

Can the chat moderator make sure nothing bad happens in the chat room?

A chat moderator supervises a chat. A moderator can kick someone out of a chat if they write something they shouldn't, but the moderator cannot stop you from going to a private chat area with someone who might harm or threaten you. If you are allowed to go to a chat, be careful to check out the topic first. Your parents/guardians can check out the chat room first to make sure the conversation is okay. Some people who go into chats may want to imagine that you are someone you are not or play out their fantasy by saying bad things to you. If anyone makes you feel uncomfortable, leave the chat immediately.

Safe Blogging

Is it safe to post a profile on MySpace, Friendster, or Facebook?

Many young people think the information they post on social networking sites such as MySpace, Friendster, or Facebook will only be seen by their friends; often, this is not the case. Anything you post on a social networking site, even if it is in a "private" area, can be seen by almost anyone, including your parents/guardians, your teachers, employers, and strangers, some of whom could be dangerous. For this reason, you should not post information about yourself. Even information that seems harmless, such as where you went to dinner last night, could be used by a stranger to find you.

You should also be careful when looking through networking sites. Scam artists have been known to use personal information from your profile to pose as a friend, in hopes that you will give them personal information, such as your credit card or cell phone numbers. Never give out any personal information online. Here are some tips to follow:

- **Before joining a social networking site, think about who might be able to see your profile.** Some sites will let only certain users see your posted content; others let everyone see postings.

- **Think about keeping some control over the information you post.** If you can, limit access to your page to a select group of people such as your friends from school, your club, your team, your community groups, or your family. Keep in mind, though, this does not always mean that other people cannot see your page.

- **Keep your information to yourself.** Do not post your full name, social security number, address, phone number, or bank and credit card account numbers, and do not post other people's information either. Be careful about posting information that could be used to identify you or locate you offline. This could include the name of your school, sports team, clubs, and where you work or hang out.

- **Make sure your screen name does not say too much about you.** Do not use your name, your age, or your hometown. It does not take a genius to combine clues to figure out who you are and where you can be found.

- **Post only information that you are comfortable with others seeing, and knowing, about you.** Many people can see your page, including your parents/guardians, your teachers, the police, the college you might want to apply to next year, or the job you might want to apply for in five years.

- **Remember that once you post information online, you cannot take it back.** Even if you delete the information from a site, older versions exist on other people's computers.

☞ Remember!!

Do not post your photo on the internet or send it to someone you do not know.

Do not post or send personal information including the following:

- full name

- address

- phone number

- login name, IM screen name, passwords

- school name

- school location

- sports teams

- clubs

- city you live in

- social security number

- financial information (credit card numbers and bank account numbers)

- where you work or hang out

- names of family members

Source: Excerpted from "Safe blogging," GirlsHealth.gov.

- **Do not post your photo.** It can be changed and spread around in ways you may not be happy about.

- **Do not flirt with strangers online.** Because some people lie about whom they really are, you never really know whom you are dealing with.

- **Do not meet someone you met online in person.** If someone you met online wants to meet you in person, tell your parents/guardians or a trusted adult right away.

- **Trust your gut if you have suspicions.** If you feel threatened by someone or uncomfortable because of something online, tell your parents/guardians or an adult you trust and report it to the police and the website. You could end up protecting someone else.

Is it okay to share my password with my best friend?

No. You should not share your password with any of your friends, even your best friend. The only people who should know your internet or e-mail password are your parents/guardians and you. If you let someone else know what your password is, then they can read anything that you may want to keep private. Another person could use bad language or go to sites you should not be visiting under your name.

Is there anything that I shouldn't tell someone on the internet?

Yes. Just like you would not walk up to a stranger and give out your phone number or share your name, where you live, or where you go to school, you should not share this kind of information online either. It is very important that you do not e-mail or IM anyone that you do not know or share any information that can identify you.

Chapter 49

Your Legal Rights As A Victim Of Sexual Assault Or Domestic Abuse

Federal Law: Domestic Abuse And Sexual Assault

All jurisdictions in the United States have laws designed to protect female victims of violence. In 1994, Congress passed the 1994 Crime Bill. A part of that crime bill package, signed into law by President Bill Clinton, was the Violence Against Women Act (VAWA). This civil rights statute, reauthorized in 1996, strengthens many of these protections and outlines federal and state enforcement provisions and penalties. VAWA strengthened prevention and prosecution of violent crimes against women and children and made domestic violence a civil rights violation. Thus, a victim of "crimes of violence motivated by gender" can bring a suit for damages in civil court and ask for restitution in criminal court. Some of the new provisions of VAWA include the following:

- greater penalties for sex crimes

- funding for programs for victims of child abuse, for the homeless, for runaways, and for street youth at risk of abuse

About This Chapter: Information in this chapter is excerpted from *Silence Hurts: Alcohol Abuse and Violence Against Women*, Prevention Pathways Online Course, Center for Substance Abuse Prevention, Substance Abuse and Mental Health Administration, U.S. Department of Health and Human Services, 2004.

- funding for states to improve law enforcement, prosecution, and services for female victims of violent crimes

- creation of a national domestic violence hotline

- denial of firearm ownership to anyone who has a civil protection order against them

- disallowing the use of past sexual behavior or alleged sexual predisposition as evidence against the victim in civil or criminal court

- requiring that the U.S. Postal Service protect the confidentiality of shelters and individual abuse victims by not disclosing addresses or other identifying information

In 2000, Congress followed up by passing VAWA II. The Violence Against Women Act II provided for a continuation of services, programs, and the creation of innovative practices and procedures begun under VAWA I. In addition, VAWA II expanded the reach of those who could be covered under its auspices to include the elderly, dating relationships and the schools, and immigrant communities.

Legal Remedies Within States

Civil Protection Orders

No consistent legal definition of domestic violence is used in every state. Each state can decide to include some people (e.g., married couples) and not others (e.g., dating couples). All states have some legal protection for victims of domestic violence.

Civil protection orders are legally binding orders designed to prevent partner abuse. The abusive partner is not allowed to contact the person at any place that she designates (e.g., home, work, school). If there are any children, their school or day care addresses would also be a place that the abuser would not be able to go to. He also cannot contact the person in any way. This would include by phone, fax, e-mail, beeper, or through another intermediary. An individual who violates such an order may face civil contempt, misdemeanor, or felony charges.

Civil protection orders are now available to battered women in every state and the District of Columbia. They are available, primarily, to prevent the abuser from continuing to abuse the victim, from having any contact with the victim, and providing the victim and her children emergency relief. For intimate partner violence and dating violence, each state has its own laws regarding civil protective orders (also called restraining orders or "no contact orders") and ex parte orders.

✔ **Quick Tip**

Local domestic violence or victim assistance centers can provide information regarding the laws in your state. To locate your state's resources or local coalitions against domestic violence, you can go to www.ndvh.org or www.vaw.umn.edu/Final Documents/FFCMatr fin.htm.

A woman who is victimized is eligible for special treatment under the law including removal of the abuser from her home (ex parte and protective orders). Although each state may differ slightly in terms of whom they consider "victims," generally, eligible victims include the following:

- a current or ex-spouse

- a co-habitant (someone who has lived in the same dwelling as a sexual partner for at least 90 days in the past 365 days)

- a child (in 75 percent of states)

- a person related to the abuser by blood, marriage, or adoption

- a parent or stepparent who has resided with the abuser for 90 days within the past year

- a "vulnerable adult" (an adult who lacks the physical or mental capacity to ensure her well being or to care for daily needs)

- an individual with a child in common with the abuser, such as a girlfriend

Some states also include dating relationships. The list above is a general representation only, and is not meant to represent any state in particular.

Prohibited Behavior

Each state has interpreted the penal code to cover various acts that would be prohibited under a civil protection order. General conduct sufficient to support the issuance of a civil protection order includes the following:

- criminal acts (such as battery, robbery, burglary, kidnapping, reckless endangerment, and criminal trespass)

- sexual assault and marital rape

- interference with personal liberty

- interference with child custody

- assaults involving motor vehicles

- harassing behaviors, stalking

- emotional abuse

- damage to property

Some states like Rhode Island, for example, prohibit any abuse, which they define as "attempting to cause or causing physical harm; placing another in fear of imminent serious physical harm; causing another to engage involuntarily in sexual relations by force, threat of force, or duress." Pennsylvania adds to its list acts that inflict false imprisonment and the physical or sexual harm of children.

Two-thirds of states allow women to file for a civil protection order "pro se"—without having to hire an attorney. Most states mandate that the courts develop special, simplified forms and instructions; provide clerical assistance for advocates; eliminate or waive initial filing fees; and provide prompt service and immediate access to the courts. Roughly half of the states allow for 24-hour access for protection orders. Some offer after-hours and weekend accessibility. In all jurisdictions except two, an abused person can obtain an ex parte temporary order of protection—often the same day the petition was filed. Most states also require that a court date is set within a specified period of time, typically between 10 and 30 days.

Nearly every state requires that all pleadings and orders filed with the court after the domestic violence incident must be served upon the defendant in a timely manner. Some states deem the defendant's appearance in court and receipt of the order as sufficient. Others require law enforcement personnel to deliver, or to make a concerted effort to deliver, the papers directly to the partner (defendant).

Ex Parte Order

Ex parte simply means "one party." In this case, the petitioner (woman) goes before a judge to obtain short-term relief. When this is granted, the abuser (respondent) may be ordered to do the following:

- refrain from further abuse

- refrain from contacting, attempting to contact, or harassing the victim

- refrain from entering the residence or workplace of the victim

- vacate the residence if the two parties were cohabitating

- remain away from the work, school, child care facility, or temporary residence of the victim or home of other family members

- give up temporary custody of a minor child

In most jurisdictions, the standard of proof required for ex parte relief is good, reasonable, or probable cause to believe that the petitioner (woman) or a member of her household is in danger of being abused or threatened with abuse by the respondent (man). The time frame for ex parte orders differs from state to state, but all states have a time limit. Some limit it to seven to ten days and others until the date of the hearing. New Jersey code specifies that a temporary restraining order remain in effect until the court takes further action.

States have all constructed their own consequences for violating an ex parte order. California's, which has among the broadest consequences, stipulates the following:

- The court can grant the requested relief for up to three years without further notice to the defendant if he does not appear at the court hearing specified on the order.

- The defendant also is notified that the abused person may obtain a more permanent restraining order when the court opens (if the ex parte order was received after hours), and that the defendant and abused should seek counsel promptly.

The order employed by the State of Rhode Island gives notice at the top of its form. It states that if a defendant violates the order, he may be guilty of a misdemeanor and can be punished by a fine or as much as a year in jail. He also may be ordered to attend counseling. Under the civil protection order, a woman can receive "emergency relief" which might include assistance in paying mortgages, childcare, car payments, or food for the children.

In 27 States, once the notice is served and the hearing is held, the length of the protection order is not to exceed one year. In Illinois and Wisconsin, the maximum duration is two years; in California and Hawaii, it is 3 years. State codes give the courts discretion to extend the duration of the order; and in some states, a violation must have occurred for an extension to be granted.

Enforcement Of Orders

Although most state codes direct that there be a system for verifying valid protection orders, some are silent about whether an officer must verify the existence of a valid order before taking any action to enforce it or to make an arrest. Roughly one-third of states mandate law enforcement officers to effect warrant-less arrests when they have probable cause to believe that a person constrained by a protection order has violated it.

> ❖ **It's A Fact!!**
> In more than 35 states, violation of a protection order constitutes a misdemeanor. In some states, violation of certain provisions of the protection order is a misdemeanor; in other states, it may only be contempt.

More than half of the states consider a violation to be a civil contempt or misdemeanor; only 21 consider a violation of the protection order criminal contempt. Mandatory counseling for the batterer is often included in the sentencing after a protection order has been violated. Some states provide a minimum jail term for violation. However, most states give the court discretion with sentencing including authorizing a maximum period of imprisonment, often for six months or one year, and a maximum fine, frequently $1,000. The purpose of the jail time or fine is for civil contempt, not criminal.

The usefulness of protection orders depends both on the specificity of the relief ordered and the enforcement practices of the police and the courts. For orders to be effective, they must be comprehensive and crafted in each case to the safety needs of the victim. A civil or criminal court may issue protective orders, either independently, or as part of a divorce or criminal complaint. They may be separate from support or child custody orders.

Police Arrests

Statutes in 47 states and the District of Columbia now authorize or mandate warrant-less, probable cause arrest, for crimes involving domestic violence. This warrant-less arrest refers to situations when police have been called to a residence in response to a 911 call. If the officer has probable cause to believe that any form of domestic violence has been committed in the home, he or she has the authority to immediately arrest the perpetrator.

Most of the state codes that have warrant-less or probable cause arrests also have a provision to notify the victim of the availability of protection orders, shelter or other emergency facilities, transportation, and sometimes even the right to file a criminal complaint.

The Massachusetts code may be the most extensive example. Beyond advising victims of the right to obtain a protection order, the code states the following:

> "You have the right to go to court and seek a criminal complaint for threats, assault and battery, assault with a deadly weapon, assault with the intent to kill, or other related offenses. If you are in need of medical treatment, you have the right to request that an officer present drive you to the nearest hospital or otherwise assist you in obtaining medical treatment."

Some states permit or mandate police officers to seize weapons used in the crime for which any probable cause misdemeanor arrest is made.

A woman may decide to file criminal charges against the perpetrator after she takes care of her immediate safety and files for a protection order. Most victim advocate centers have attorneys available (or know some in the community) to help women work through the legal process of filing criminal charges, which may include assault, assault and battery, sexual assault, or assault with the intent to kill.

Batterer Intervention Services

Almost half of the states in the country have adopted codes that address providing treatment or educational services for abusive men. Most states do not fund batterer programs, instead requiring that each man pay a nominal fee for the service.

Some states, like Arizona, Connecticut, and California, either require pre-trial counseling, or use it as an option for pre-trial diversion for offenders who have not previously participated in a family violence education program or other accelerated rehabilitation and who are charged with misdemeanors.

Most states authorizing court-ordered intervention services do so in the civil protection order. Courts may choose among different programs and treatment modalities available in that geographic area. Washington State has the most comprehensive code regarding batterer's intervention and other necessities for batterer programs.

Filing A Civil Lawsuit

> ♣ **It's A Fact!!**
> Criminal codes require specialized treatment programs designed especially for men who batter their wives or partners.

Any crime victim can file a civil lawsuit against a perpetrator, regardless of the outcome of any criminal prosecution and without any criminal proceeding. In a civil case, an abuser is called the defendant. Unlike the criminal justice process, the civil justice system does not attempt to determine whether the defendant is guilty or innocent. Defendants are not put in prison. Rather, civil courts attempt to determine whether a defendant or a third party is liable for the injuries sustained as a result of the crime. If the defendant is found liable in this civil process, he probably will have to pay monetary damages to the victim.

When building a civil case, the victim must make the effort to provide the court or an attorney the following facts:

- date and time of criminal act

- location of events, addresses, and description of premises

- whether a police report was filed, and if so, identification of the police department where the complaint was filed, the officer or detective who took the complaint, the report number, and any statements taken as part of an investigation

- anyone who might have seen the crime

- whether there was a criminal case, and if so, the identification of the prosecutor, current status of the case, and a description of the facts of the case

- any available information about the perpetrator including name, address, social security number, any aliases, employment information, any assets and insurance coverage, physical description, and any identifying features

- a listing of the physical, emotional, and psychological injuries that resulted from the assault and the cost of anticipated treatment

- information about any property damage and how much time and money the victim lost from her job

The decision to press charges is difficult but significant. As more courts and communities are forced to deal with rape and abuse, awareness about these crimes will increase, and women can claim the right to have these concerns taken seriously.

A woman may decide to drop the civil charges because she does not want her personal life aired publicly. Sometimes there might be educational, age, or economic barriers to pursuing a case. Some women might not want family or friends to know about the rape or assault. Some women avoid pressing charges because they fear retaliation. However, repeat rapes are uncommon, even in cases when a rapist threatens to return if he is reported.

Chapter 50

Bullying And The Law

Federal Law

Compared with European countries, the United States has been slow to respond to school bullying. However, several laws have been passed over the last several years that require states to take action to curb bullying behaviors.

The No Child Left Behind (NCLB) Act of 2001, Title 20 (Education), contains a drug and violence prevention component under Safe and Drug-Free Schools and Communities (Title IV). The NCLB Act retains state formula grants already in existence and national discretionary activities for drug and violence prevention. It also does the following:

- Allows a student in a persistently dangerous school, or a student who is victimized at school, to transfer to a safe school.

- Requires states to report on school safety to the public.

- Requires school districts to implement drug and violence prevention programs of demonstrated effectiveness.

About This Chapter: Information in this chapter is excerpted from *The ABCs of Bullying: Addressing, Blocking, and Curbing School Aggression*, Prevention Pathways Online Course, Center for Substance Abuse Prevention, Substance Abuse and Mental Health Administration, U.S. Department of Health and Human Services, 2004.

- Requires local education agencies (LEAs) that receive Safe and Drug-Free Schools moneys to have a detailed plan for keeping schools safe. The plan must include the following:

  1. Appropriate and effective discipline policies

  2. Security procedures

  3. Prevention activities

  4. A student code of conduct

  5. A crisis management plan for responding to violent or traumatic incidents on school property

> ♣ **It's A Fact!!**
> The U.S. Supreme Court has clearly stated that a school district is liable if administrators knew, or should have known, that bullying (some methods legally termed harassment) was occurring and failed to take immediate and appropriate action.

In addition, the NCLB Act made specific requirement changes to the Safe and Drug-Free Schools and Communities program addressing the following:

- Mandating community service for expelled or suspended students

- Creating a school security and technology resource center

- Creating a national center for school and youth safety to do the following:

  1. Provide emergency counseling, enhanced security assistance, and a toll-free hotline for students to report violence and/or criminal activity

  2. Provide information and outreach (best practices, clearinghouse for model school safety programs, etc.)

- Creating a Safe and Drug-Free Schools and Communities Advisory Committee

- Mandating a detailed local plan for Safe and Drug-Free Schools

In the context of sexual bullying, the Office of Civil Rights (OCR) has passed comprehensive policies prohibiting discrimination within all programs and activities. OCR enforces Title IX, which prohibits discrimination based on a student's sex in schools receiving federal funds.

Federal Initiatives

In recognition of the magnitude of the problem, as well as schools' responsibility to provide a safe learning environment for students, the U.S. Government has launched a multiyear public education campaign on bullying.

The Bullying Prevention Campaign uses a variety of communications messages to help prevent bullying. In keeping with the practice of leaving states responsible for education, the U.S. government does not dictate specific laws relating to bullying for all states, but leaves it up to each state to pass its own legislation. However, all states are required to provide all students with an accessible, competent, and safe learning environment.

State Laws

How do states adapt the federal requirements under the Safe and Drug-Free Schools provision? Many states have taken legislative action to stop bullying, harassment, and hate crimes. Most of the legislative responses require the state's Department of Education, school districts, and school boards to develop policies and procedures to prevent bullying. Most of the state laws cover bullying that occurs on school grounds and at school-sponsored activities.

Unfortunately, there is no national mandated and uniform school crime reporting to help schools assess issues and concerns. Only a little more than a dozen states now require crime reporting in grades K–2. One of the reasons that national legislation has not been developed is that educators do not like to report problems and deficiencies that may exist on their campuses.

The National Conference of State Legislatures has compiled a list of state actions that relate to bullying, harassment, and hate crimes. States that have passed formal laws on bullying include California, Colorado, Connecticut, Georgia, Illinois, Louisiana, Mississippi, Nevada, New Hampshire, New Jersey, Oklahoma, Oregon, Vermont, Washington, and West Virginia. For more information, contact the National Conference of State Legislatures (http://www.ncsl.org) or http://www.bullypolice.org.

Part Five

If You Need More Information

Chapter 51

Abuse And Violence: A Statistical Summary

Child Maltreatment Facts

Occurrence

- Data on the confirmed number of U.S. child maltreatment cases in 2002 are available from child protective service agencies, but these data are generally considered underestimates:

  - Child protective service agencies confirmed that 906,000 children were maltreated in the United States.

  - Among children confirmed by child protective service agencies as being maltreated, 61% experienced neglect; 19% were physically abused; 10% were sexually abused; and 5% were emotionally or psychologically abused.

  - An estimated 1,500 children were confirmed to have died from maltreatment; 36% of these deaths were from neglect, 28% from physical abuse, and 29% from multiple maltreatment types.

About This Chapter: Information in this chapter is from "Child Maltreatment: Fact Sheet," September 2006, "Intimate Partner Violence: Fact Sheet," October 2006, "Sexual Violence: Fact Sheet," September 2006, and "Youth Violence: Fact Sheet," September 2006, National Center for Injury Prevention and Control, Centers for Disease Control and Prevention.

- Shaken-baby syndrome (SBS) is a form of child abuse affecting between 1,200 and 1,600 children every year. SBS is a collection of signs and symptoms resulting from violently shaking an infant or child.

Consequences

- Children who experience maltreatment are at increased risk for adverse health effects and behaviors as adults including smoking, alcoholism, drug abuse, eating disorders, severe obesity, depression, suicide, sexual promiscuity, and certain chronic diseases.

- Maltreatment during infancy or early childhood can cause important regions of the brain to form improperly, leading to physical, mental, and emotional problems such as sleep disturbances, panic disorder, and attention-deficit/hyperactivity disorder.

- About 25% to 30% of infant victims with SBS die from their injuries. Nonfatal consequences of SBS include varying degrees of visual impairment (e.g., blindness), motor impairment (e.g. cerebral palsy), and cognitive impairments.

- Victims of child maltreatment who were physically assaulted by caregivers are twice as likely to be physically assaulted as adults.

- Direct costs (judicial, law enforcement, and health system responses to child maltreatment) are estimated at $24 billion each year. The indirect costs (long-term economic consequences of child maltreatment) exceed an estimated $69 billion annually.

Groups At Risk

- Children younger than four years are at greatest risk of severe injury or death. In 2003, children younger than four years accounted for 79% of child maltreatment fatalities, with infants under one year accounting for 44% of deaths.

Risk And Protective Factors

A combination of individual, relational, community, and societal factors contribute to the risk of child maltreatment. Although children are not responsible for the harm inflicted upon them, certain individual characteristics have been found to increase their risk of being maltreated. Risk factors are contributing factors—not direct causes.

Examples of risk factors are as follows:

- disabilities or mental retardation in children that may increase caregiver burden

- social isolation of families

- parents' lack of understanding of children's needs and child development

♣ It's A Fact!!

Children who experience maltreatment are at increased risk for adverse health effects and behaviors as adults including smoking, alcoholism, drug abuse, eating disorders, severe obesity, depression, suicide, sexual promiscuity, and certain chronic diseases.

Source: Excerpted from "Child Maltreatment: Fact Sheet," National Center for Injury Prevention and Control, Centers for Disease Control and Prevention.

- parents' history of domestic abuse

- poverty and other socioeconomic disadvantage, such as unemployment

- family disorganization, dissolution, and violence including intimate partner violence

- lack of family cohesion

- substance abuse in family

- young, single non-biological parents

- poor parent-child relationships and negative interactions

- parental thoughts and emotions supporting maltreatment behaviors

- parental stress and distress including depression or other mental health conditions

- community violence

Protective factors are the opposite of risk factors and may lessen the risk of child maltreatment. Protective factors exist at individual, relational, community, and societal levels.

Examples of protective factors are as follows:

- supportive family environment

- nurturing parenting skills

- stable family relationships

- household rules and monitoring of the child

- parental employment

- adequate housing

- access to health care and social services

- caring adults outside family who can serve as role models or mentors

- communities that support parents and take responsibility for preventing abuse

Intimate Partner Violence Facts

Occurrence

Statistics about intimate partner violence (IPV) vary because of differences in how different data sources define IPV and collect data. For example, some definitions include stalking and psychological abuse, and others consider only physical and sexual violence. Data on IPV usually come from police, clinical settings, nongovernmental organizations, and survey research.

Most IPV incidents are not reported to the police. About 20% of IPV rapes or sexual assaults, 25% of physical assaults, and 50% of stalkings directed toward women are reported. Even fewer IPV incidents against men are reported. Thus, it is believed that available data greatly underestimate the true magnitude of the problem. While not an exhaustive list, here are some statistics on the occurrence of IPV. In many cases, the severity of the IPV behaviors is unknown.

- Nearly 5.3 million incidents of IPV occur each year among U.S. women ages 18 and older, and 3.2 million occur among men. Most assaults are relatively minor and consist of pushing, grabbing, shoving, slapping, and hitting.

- In the United States every year, about 1.5 million women and more than 800,000 men are raped or physically assaulted by an intimate partner. This translates into about 47 IPV assaults per 1,000 women and 32 assaults per 1,000 men.

- IPV results in nearly 2 million injuries and 1,300 deaths nationwide every year.

- Estimates indicate more than 1 million women and 371,000 men are stalked by intimate partners each year.

- IPV accounted for 20% of nonfatal violence against women in 2001 and 3% against men.

- From 1976 to 2002, about 11% of homicide victims were killed by an intimate partner.

- In 2002, 76% of IPV homicide victims were female; 24% were male.

- The number of intimate partner homicides decreased 14% overall for men and women in the span of about 20 years, with a 67% decrease for men (from 1,357 to 388) vs. 25% for women (from 1,600 to 1,202).

- One study found that 44% of women murdered by their intimate partner had visited an emergency department within 2 years of the homicide. Of these women, 93% had at least one injury visit.

- Previous literature suggests that women who have separated from their abusive partners often remain at risk of violence.

- Firearms were the major weapon type used in intimate partner homicides from 1981 to 1998.

- A national study found that 29% of women and 22% of men had experienced physical, sexual, or psychological IPV during their lifetime.

- Between 4% and 8% of pregnant women are abused at least once during the pregnancy.

Consequences

In general, victims of repeated violence over time experience more serious consequences than victims of one-time incidents. The following information describes just some of the consequences of IPV.

Physical: At least 42% of women and 20% of men who were physically assaulted since age 18 sustained injuries during their most recent victimization. Most injuries were minor such as scratches, bruises, and welts.

More severe physical consequences of IPV may occur depending on severity and frequency of abuse. These include the following:

- bruises

- knife wounds

- pelvic pain

- headaches

- back pain

- broken bones

- gynecological disorders

> **♣ It's A Fact!!**
>
> One study found that children of abused mothers were 57 times more likely to have been harmed because of IPV between their parents compared with children of non-abused mothers.
>
> Source: Excerpted from "Intimate Partner Violence: Fact Sheet," National Center for Injury Prevention and Control, Centers for Disease Control and Prevention.

- pregnancy difficulties like low birth weight babies and perinatal deaths

- sexually transmitted diseases including human immunodeficiency virus/ acquired immunodeficiency syndrome (HIV/AIDS)

- central nervous system disorders

- gastrointestinal disorders

- symptoms of post-traumatic stress disorder

- emotional detachment

- sleep disturbances
- flashbacks
- replaying assault in mind
- heart or circulatory conditions

Children may become injured during IPV incidents between their parents. A large overlap exists between IPV and child maltreatment.

Psychological: Physical violence is typically accompanied by emotional or psychological abuse. IPV, whether sexual, physical, or psychological, can lead to various psychological consequences for victims. These consequences are as follows:

- depression
- antisocial behavior
- suicidal behavior in females
- anxiety
- low self-esteem
- inability to trust men
- fear of intimacy

Social: Victims of IPV sometimes face the following social consequences:

- restricted access to services
- strained relationships with health providers and employers
- isolation from social networks

Health Behaviors: Women with a history of IPV are more likely to display behaviors that present further health risks (e.g., substance abuse, alcoholism, suicide attempts).

IPV is associated with a variety of negative health behaviors. Studies show that the more severe the violence, the stronger its relationship to negative health behaviors by victims.

- engaging in high-risk sexual behavior
  - unprotected sex

- decreased condom use
- early sexual initiation
- choosing unhealthy sexual partners
- having multiple sex partners
- trading sex for food, money, or other items
- using or abusing harmful substances
  - smoking cigarettes
  - drinking alcohol
  - driving after drinking alcohol
  - taking drugs
- unhealthy diet-related behaviors
  - fasting
  - vomiting
  - abusing diet pills
  - overeating
- overuse of health services

Economic: The following items illustrate the economic consequences of intimate partner violence.

- Costs of IPV against women in 1995 exceed an estimated $5.8 billion. These costs include nearly $4.1 billion in the direct costs of medical and mental health care and nearly $1.8 billion in the indirect costs of lost productivity.
- When updated to 2003 dollars, IPV costs exceed $8.3 billion, which includes $460 million for rape, $6.2 billion for physical assault, $461 million for stalking, and $1.2 billion in the value of lost lives.
- Victims of severe IPV lose nearly 8 million days of paid work, the equivalent of more than 32,000 full-time jobs, and almost 5.6 million days of household productivity each year.
- Women who experience severe aggression by men (e.g., not being allowed to go to work or school, or having their lives or their children's

lives threatened) are more likely to have been unemployed in the past, have health problems, and be receiving public assistance.

Groups At Risk

Certain groups are at greater risk for IPV victimization or perpetration.

Victimization

- The National Crime Victimization Survey found that 85% of IPV victims were women.

- Prevalence of IPV varies among race. Among the ethnic groups most at risk are American Indian/Alaskan Native women and men, African American women, and Hispanic women.

- Young women, and those below the poverty line, are disproportionately victims of IPV.

Perpetration

- Studies show that for low levels of physical violence, men and women self-report perpetrating physical IPV at about the same rate. However, a common criticism of these studies is that they are generally lacking information on the context of the violence (e.g., whether self-defense is the reason for the violence).

Risk Factors For Victimization

Individual Factors
- prior history of IPV
- being female
- young age
- heavy alcohol and drug use
- high-risk sexual behavior
- witnessing or experiencing violence as a child
- being less educated
- unemployment
- for men, having a different ethnicity from their partner's

- for women, having a greater education level than their partner's
- for women, being American Indian/Alaska Native or African American
- for women, having a verbally abusive, jealous, or possessive partner

Relationship Factors

- couples with income, educational, or job status disparities
- dominance and control of the relationship by the male

Community Factors

- poverty and associated factors (e.g., overcrowding)
- low social capital—lack of institutions, relationships, and norms that shape the quality and quantity of a community's social interactions
- weak community sanctions against IPV (e.g., police unwilling to intervene)

Societal Factors

- traditional gender norms (e.g., women should stay at home and not enter workforce, should be submissive)

Risk Factors For Perpetration

Individual Factors

- low self-esteem
- low income
- low academic achievement
- involvement in aggressive or delinquent behavior as a youth
- heavy alcohol and drug use
- depression
- anger and hostility
- personality disorders
- prior history of being physically abusive
- having few friends and being isolated from other people
- unemployment
- economic stress

- emotional dependence and insecurity
- belief in strict gender roles (e.g., male dominance and aggression in relationships)
- desire for power and control in relationships
- being a victim of physical or psychological abuse (consistently one of the strongest predictors of perpetration)

Relationship Factors

- marital conflict—fights, tension, and other struggles
- marital instability—divorces and separations
- dominance and control of the relationship by the male
- economic stress
- unhealthy family relationships and interactions

Community Factors

- poverty and associated factors (e.g., overcrowding)
- low social capital—lack of institutions, relationships, and norms that shape the quality and quantity of a community's social interactions
- weak community sanctions against IPV (e.g., unwillingness of neighbors to intervene in situations where they witness violence)

Societal Factors

- traditional gender norms (e.g., women should stay at home and not enter workforce, should be submissive)

Protective Factors

Little is known about what factors can lessen the likelihood of IPV victimization or perpetration.

Sexual Violence Facts

Occurrence

Sexual violence is a serious problem that affects millions of people every year. Its victims are at increased risk of being abused again. Sexual violence perpetrators are also at increased risk of perpetrating again.

Statistics about sexual violence vary due to differences in how it is defined and how data is collected. Sexual violence data usually come from police, clinical settings, nongovernmental organizations, and survey research.

Available data greatly underestimate the true magnitude of the problem. Rape is one of the most underreported crimes. In 2002, only 39% of rapes and sexual assaults were reported to law enforcement officials. While not an exhaustive list, here are some statistics on the occurrence of sexual violence.

- About 2 out of 1,000 children in the United States were confirmed by child protective service agencies as having experienced sexual assault in 2003.

- Among high school youth nationwide the following is true:
  - About 9% of students reported that they had been forced to have sexual intercourse.
  - Female students are more likely than male students to report sexual assault (11.9% vs. 6.1%).
  - Overall, 12.3% of African American students, 10.4% of Hispanic students, and 7.3% of White students reported that they had been forced to have sexual intercourse.

> ✤ **It's A Fact!!**
> Among high school youth nationwide, about 9% of students reported that they had been forced to have sexual intercourse.
>
> Source: Excerpted from "Sexual Violence: Fact Sheet," National Center for Injury Prevention and Control, Centers for Disease Control and Prevention.

- Among college students nationwide, between 20% and 25% of women reported experiencing completed or attempted rape.

- Among adults nationwide, the following is true:
  - More than 300,000 women (0.3%) and over 90,000 men (0.1%) reported being raped in the previous 12 months.
  - One in six women (17%) and one in thirty-three men (3%) reported experiencing an attempted or completed rape at some time in their lives.

- Rape usually occurs more than once. Among adults who report being raped, women experienced 2.9 rapes and men experienced 1.2 rapes in the previous year.

Consequences

Sexual violence can have very harmful and lasting consequences for victims, families, and communities. The following list describes just some of them.

Physical

- Women who experience both sexual and physical abuse are significantly more likely to have sexually transmitted diseases.

- Over 32,000 pregnancies result from rape every year.

- There are long-term consequences such as the following:
  - chronic pelvic pain
  - premenstrual syndrome
  - gastrointestinal disorders
  - gynecological and pregnancy complications
  - migraines and other frequent headaches
  - back pain
  - facial pain
  - disability preventing work

Psychological

Victims of sexual violence face both immediate and long-term psychological consequences.

Immediate psychological consequences include the following:

- shock
- denial
- fear
- confusion
- anxiety
- withdrawal

- guilt
- nervousness
- distrust of others
- symptoms of post-traumatic stress disorder
  - emotional detachment
  - sleep disturbances
  - flashbacks
  - mental replay of assault

Mental chronic psychological consequences include the following:

- depression
- attempted or completed suicide
- alienation
- post-traumatic stress disorder
- unhealthy diet-related behaviors
  - fasting
  - vomiting
  - abusing diet pills
  - overeating

Social

- strained relationships with the victim's family, friends, and intimate partners
- less emotional support from friends and family
- less frequent contact with friends and relatives
- lower likelihood of marriage

Health Behaviors

Some researchers view the following health behaviors as both consequences of sexual violence and factors that increase a person's vulnerability to being victimized again in the future:

> ♣ **It's A Fact!!**
> More than half of all rapes of women (54%) occur before age 18.
>
> Source: Excerpted from "Sexual Violence: Fact Sheet," National Center for Injury Prevention and Control, Centers for Disease Control and Prevention.

- engaging in high-risk sexual behavior including the following:
  - unprotected sex
  - early sexual initiation
  - choosing unhealthy sexual partners
  - having multiple sex partners
  - trading sex for food, money, or other items
- using or abusing harmful substances including the following:
  - smoking cigarettes
  - drinking alcohol
  - driving after drinking alcohol
  - taking drugs

Groups At Risk

Certain groups are at risk for IPV victimization or perpetration.

Victimization

- Women are more likely to be victims of sexual violence than men: 78% of the victims of rape and sexual assault are women and 22% are men.

- Sexual violence starts very early in life. More than half of all rapes of women (54%) occur before age 18; 22% of these rapes occur before age 12. For men, 75% of all rapes occur before age 18, and 48% occur before age 12.

- Prevalence of IPV varies among race. American Indian and Alaskan Native women are significantly more likely (34%) to report being raped than African American women (19%) or White women (18%).

- Women in college who use drugs, attend a university with high drinking rates, belong in a sorority, and drank heavily in high school are at greater risk for rape while intoxicated.

Perpetration

- Most perpetrators of sexual violence are men. Among acts of sexual violence committed against women since the age of 18, 100% of rapes,

92% of physical assaults, and 97% of stalking acts were perpetrated by men. Sexual violence against men is also mainly male violence; men perpetrated 70% of rapes, 86% of physical assaults, and 65% of stalking acts.

Relationship Between Victim And Perpetrator

- In 8 out of 10 rape cases, the victim knows the perpetrator.

- A national survey found that 10% of women were victims of rape or attempted rape by a husband or intimate partner in their lifetime.

- Of people who report sexual violence, 64% of women, and 16% of men were raped, physically assaulted, or stalked by an intimate partner. This includes a current or former spouse, cohabitating partner, boy-friend/girlfriend, or date.

Vulnerability Factors For Victimization

Populations vulnerable to victimization and those at risk for perpetration can share some factors. Shared individual-level factors are noted below with an asterisk (*).

♣ **It's A Fact!!**

In 8 out of 10 rape cases, the victim knows the perpetrator.

Source: Excerpted from "Sexual Violence: Fact Sheet," National Center for Injury Prevention and Control, Centers for Disease Control and Prevention.

- **Prior History Of Sexual Violence:** Women who are raped before the age of 18 are twice as likely to be raped as adults, compared to those without a history of sexual abuse.

- **Gender:** Women are more likely to be victims of sexual violence than men: 78% of the victims of rape and sexual assault are women and 22% are men. These findings may be influenced by the reluctance of men to report sexual violence.

- **Young Age:** Sexual violence victimization starts very early in life. More than half of all rapes of women (54%) occur before age 18; 22% of these rapes occur before age 12. For men, 75% of all rapes occur before age 18, and 48% occur before age 12. Young women are at higher risk of being raped than older women.

- **Drug Or Alcohol Use:*** Binge drinking and drug use are related to increased rates of victimization.

- **High-Risk Sexual Behavior:** As with drug/alcohol use, researchers are trying to understand the complex relationships between sexuality and sexual violence—their causality, directionality, and other etiologic factors that increase vulnerability for victimization are not well understood. Some researchers believe that engaging in high-risk sexual behavior is both a vulnerability factor and a consequence of childhood sexual abuse. Youth with many sexual partners are at increased risk of experiencing sexual abuse.

- **Poverty:*** Poverty may make the daily lives of women and children more dangerous (e.g. walking alone at night, less parental supervision). It may also make them more dependent on men for survival, and therefore, less able to control their own sexuality, consent to sex, recognize their own victimization, or to seek help when victimized. These issues increase their vulnerability to sexual victimization. In addition, poor women may be at risk for sexual violence because their economic (and, often, educational) status necessitates that they engage in high-risk survival activities, for example trading sex for food, money, or other items. Poverty also puts women at increased risk of intimate partner violence, of which sexual violence is often one aspect.

- **Ethnicity/Culture:** American Indian and Alaskan Native women are more likely (34%) to report being raped than African American women (19%), White women (18%), or Hispanic women (15%).

Risk Factors For Perpetration

Individual Factors

- alcohol and drug use*
- coercive sexual fantasies
- impulsive and antisocial tendencies
- preference for impersonal sex
- hostility towards women

- hypermasculinity
- childhood history of sexual and physical abuse*
- witnessed family violence as a child

Relationship Factors

- association with sexually aggressive and delinquent peers
- family environment characterized by physical violence and few resources
- strong patriarchal relationship or familial environment
- emotionally unsupportive familial environment

Community Factors

- lack of employment opportunities
- lack of institutional support from police and judicial system
- general tolerance of sexual assault within the community
- settings that support sexual violence
- weak community sanctions against sexual violence perpetrators

Societal Factors

- poverty
- societal norms that support sexual violence
- societal norms that support male superiority and sexual entitlement
- societal norms that maintain women's inferiority and sexual submissiveness
- weak laws and policies related to gender equity
- high tolerance levels of crime and other forms of violence

Protective Factors

Protective factors may lessen the likelihood of sexual violence victimization or perpetration and exist at individual, relational, community, and societal levels. Although less is known about protective factors, the literature suggests measures to prevent potential perpetrators. Some examples for youth are connectedness with school, friends, and adults in the community, and emotional health.

Youth Violence Facts

Occurrence

Youth violence is an important public health problem that results in deaths and injuries. The following statistics provide an overview of youth violence in the United States:

- In 2003, 5,570 young people ages 10 to 24 were murdered—an average of 15 each day. Of these victims, 82% were killed with firearms.

- Although high-profile school shootings have increased public concern for student safety, school-associated violent deaths account for less than 1% of homicides among school-aged children and youth.

- In 2004, more than 750,000 young people ages 10 to 24 were treated in emergency departments for injuries sustained due to violence.

- In a nationwide survey of high school students, the following was found to be true:

  - Thirty-three percent reported being in a physical fight one or more times in the 12 months preceding the survey.

  - Seventeen percent reported carrying a weapon (e.g., gun, knife, or club) on one or more of the 30 days preceding the survey.

- An estimated 30% of 6th to 10th graders in the United States were involved in bullying as a bully, a target of bullying, or both.

Consequences

- Direct and indirect costs of youth violence (e.g., medical, lost productivity, quality of life) exceed $158 billion every year.

- In a nationwide survey of high school students, about 6% reported not going to school on one or more days in the 30 days preceding the survey, because they felt unsafe at school or on their way to and from school.

- In addition to causing injury and death, youth violence affects communities by increasing the cost of health care, reducing productivity, decreasing property values, and disrupting social services.

Groups At Risk

- Among 10 to 24 year olds, homicide is the leading cause of death for African Americans, the second leading cause of death for Hispanics, and the third leading cause of death for American Indians, Alaska Natives, and Asian/Pacific Islanders.

- Of the 5,570 homicides reported in 2003 among 10 to 24 year olds, 86% were males and 14% were females.

- Male students are more likely to be involved in a physical fight than female students (41% vs. 25%).

Risk Factors

Research on youth violence has increased our understanding of factors that make some populations more vulnerable to victimization and perpetration. Many risk factors are the same, in part, because of the overlap among victims and perpetrators of violence.

Risk factors increase the likelihood that a young person will become violent. However, risk factors are not direct causes of youth violence; instead, risk factors contribute to youth violence.

Individual Risk Factors

- history of violent victimization or involvement
- attention deficits, hyperactivity, or learning disorders
- history of early aggressive behavior
- involvement with drugs, alcohol, or tobacco
- low IQ
- poor behavioral control
- deficits in social cognitive or information-processing abilities
- high emotional distress
- history of treatment for emotional problems
- antisocial beliefs and attitudes
- exposure to violence and conflict in the family

Family Risk Factors

- authoritarian childrearing attitudes
- harsh, lax, or inconsistent disciplinary practices
- low parental involvement
- low emotional attachment to parents or caregivers
- low parental education and income
- parental substance abuse or criminality
- poor family functioning
- poor monitoring and supervision of children

Peer/School Risk Factors

- association with delinquent peers
- involvement in gangs
- social rejection by peers
- lack of involvement in conventional activities
- poor academic performance
- low commitment to school and school failure

♣ It's A Fact!!

Although high-profile school shootings have increased public concern for student safety, school-associated violent deaths account for less than 1% of homicides among school-aged children and youth.

Source: Excerpted from "Youth Violence: Fact Sheet," National Center for Injury Prevention and Control, Centers for Disease Control and Prevention.

Community Risk Factors

- diminished economic opportunities
- high concentrations of poor residents
- high level of transiency
- high level of family disruption
- low levels of community participation
- socially disorganized neighborhoods

Protective Factors

Protective factors buffer young people from risks of becoming violent. These factors exist at various levels. To date, protective factors have not been studied as extensively or rigorously as risk factors. However, identifying and understanding protective factors are equally as important as researching risk factors.

Individual Protective Factors

- intolerant attitude toward deviance
- high IQ or high grade point average
- positive social orientation
- religiosity

Family Protective Factors

- connectedness to family or adults outside of the family
- ability to discuss problems with parents
- perceived parental expectations about school performance are high
- frequent shared activities with parents
- consistent presence of parent during at least one of the following: when awakening, when arriving home from school, at evening mealtime, and when going to bed
- involvement in social activities

Peer/School Protective Factors

- commitment to school
- involvement in social activities

Chapter 52

Directory Of Abuse And Violence Resources

Teen Dating Violence Resource List

Hotlines

National Domestic Violence Hotline, 24 hours, 1-800-799-SAFE (7233), 1-800-787-3224 (TTY): The National Domestic Violence Hotline links individuals to help in their area using a nationwide database that includes detailed information on domestic violence shelters, other emergency shelters, legal advocacy and assistance programs, and social service programs.

National Hopeline Network, 24 hours, 1-800-SUICIDE (784-2433): The National Hopeline Network provides suicide, crisis, and domestic violence service referrals for teens. Callers are automatically routed to the closest certified crisis center.

National Runaway Hotline, 24 hours, 1-800-Runaway, 1-800-621-0394 (TDD): The National Runaway Switchboard operates a confidential hotline

About This Chapter: Information under the heading "Teen Dating Violence Resource List" is reprinted with permission from the Family Violence Prevention Fund, www.endabuse.org. Copyright © 2007 Family Violence Prevention Fund. All rights reserved. Text under the heading "Additional Abuse And Violence Resources" is excerpted from *Use of Computers in the Sexual Exploitation of Children, Second Edition*, by Daniel S. Armagh and Nick L. Battaglia, Office of Juvenile Justice and Delinquency Prevention, Office of Justice Programs, U.S. Department of Justice, December 2006. All contact information was verified in May 2007.

for runaway youth, teens in crisis, and concerned friends and family members. All services are free and available 24 hours every day. Website: www.nrscrisisline.org.

Rape Abuse and Incest National Network (RAINN), 24 hours, 1-800-656-HOPE: The Rape, Abuse, Incest National Network will automatically transfer the caller to the nearest rape crisis center anywhere in the nation. It can be used as a last resort if people cannot find a domestic violence shelter.

Domestic Violence Organizations

Family Violence Prevention Fund (FVPF) is a national nonprofit organization that focuses on domestic violence education, prevention, and public policy reform. Address: 383 Rhode Island Street, Suite 304, San Francisco, CA 94103-5133, Phone: 415-252-8900, Fax: 415-252-8991, E-mail: fund@fvpf.org, Website: www.fvpf.org.

The National Health Resource Center on Domestic Violence, a project of the FVPF, provides support to thousands of health care professionals, policy makers, and domestic violence advocates through its four main program areas: model training strategies, practical tools, technical assistance, and public policy. Phone: 888-Rx-ABUSE, Fax: 415-252-8991, E-mail: health@fvpf.org, Website: www.fvpf.org/health.

National Coalition Against Domestic Violence (NCADV) is dedicated to the empowerment of battered women and their children and therefore is committed to the elimination of personal and societal violence in the lives of battered women and their children. Teen Dating Violence Project, Address: PO Box 18749, Denver, CO 80218, Phone: 303-839-1852, Fax: 303-831-9251, Website: www.ncadv.org.

Pennsylvania Coalition Against Domestic Violence and National Resource Center (PCADV) is a private, nonprofit membership organization and is dedicated to ending domestic violence and helping battered women and their children reestablish physical, social, and economic dignity. Address: 6400 Flank Drive, Suite 1300, Harrisburg, PA 17112, Phone: 800-932-4632, Fax: 717-671-8149, Website: www.pcadv.org.

Teen Dating Violence

Break the Cycle is a national nonprofit organization whose mission is to engage, educate, and empower youth to build lives and communities free from dating and domestic violence. Address: PO Box 64996, Los Angeles, CA 90064, Phone: 888-988-TEEN, E-mail: info@breakthecycle.org, Website: www.breakthecycle.org.

The Empower Program works with youth to end the culture of violence. Address: 1312 8th Street, Washington, DC 20001, Fax: 202-234-1901, E-mail: empower@empowered.org, Website: www.empowered.org.

Girls Incorporated National Resource Center is a national youth organization dedicated to inspiring all girls to be strong, smart, and bold. Address: 441 West Michigan Street, Indianapolis, IN 46202, Phone: 317-634-7546, Fax: 317-634-3024, E-mail: girlsinc@girls-inc.org, Website: www.girlsinc.org.

Liz Claiborne Inc. produces "A Teen's Handbook" and web pages to help teens learn about dating violence by providing facts, guidance, and resources. To order a free handbook, Phone: 800-449-STOP (7867), Website: www.lizclaiborne.com/lizinc/lizworks/women/handbook.asp#teen.

Los Angeles Commission on Assaults Against Women (LACAAW) is a nonprofit, multi-cultural, community-based organization whose mission is the elimination of violence against women, youth, and children. The In Touch With Teens Program provides education, training, and technical assistance to youth and service providers on preventing dating violence. Address: 605 West Olympic Boulevard, Suite 400, Los Angeles, CA 90015, Phone: 213-955-9090, Hotline: 213-626-3393, TTY: 213-955-9095, Fax: 213-955-9093, E-mail: info@lacaaw.org, Website: www.lacaaw.org.

SafeNetwork is a project of the California Department of Health Services, California District Attorneys Association. SafeNetwork maintains comprehensive materials and information for both teens and service providers including a teen safety plan, directory of shelters, technical assistance, and training information. Address: PO Box 161810, Austin, Texas 78716, 1-800-799-SAFE, Website: www.safenetwork.net/teens/teens.html.

Lesbian, Gay, Bisexual, Transgendered, Queer (LGBTQ) Youth

Community United Against Violence (CUAV) is a 20-year-old multicultural organization working to end violence against and within lesbian, gay, bisexual, transgender, and queer/questioning (LGBTQ) communities. The Love and Justice Project aims to lead the discussion on positive communication skills, consensual sexuality, partnership decision making, and naming abusive behavior in LGBTQ youth relationships by building bridges and community resources between LGBTQ youth and elders. Address: 170A Cap Street, San Francisco, CA 94110, Phone: 415-777-5500, Fax: 415-777-5565, 24 Hour Support Line: 415-333-HELP (4357), E-mail: cuav@aol.com, Website: www.cuav.org.

Parents, Families, and Friends of Lesbians and Gays (PFLAG) is a national organization that promotes the health and well-being of gay, lesbian, bisexual and transgendered persons, their families, and friends. Their website provides users with information on local chapters, advocacy and support information, and other resources that support the family and friends of gays and lesbians. Address: 1726 M Street, NW, Suite 400, Washington, DC 20036, Phone: 202-467-8180, Fax: 202-467-8194, E-mail: info@pflag.org, Website: www.pflag.org.

Teen Pregnancy

American College of Obstetricians and Gynecologists (ACOG) has a membership of 40,000 physicians and is the nation's leading group of professionals providing health care for women. ACOG's website provides adolescent sexual assault screening tools as well as other teen pregnancy materials. To request free copies of their educational bulletins, Phone: 202-638-5577 or E-mail: violence@acog.org. Address: ACOG, 409 12th Street, SW, Washington, DC 20024, PO Box 96920, Washington, DC 20090, Phone: 202-863-2487, Fax: 202-484-3917, E-mail: adolhlth@acog.org, Website: www.acog.org.

Sexual Assault

Center for the Prevention of Sexual and Domestic Violence is an inter-religious educational resource addressing issues of sexual and domestic violence whose goal is to engage religious leaders in the task of ending abuse and to serve as a bridge between religious and secular communities. Their emphasis is on education and prevention. Address: 2400 North 34th Street, Suite 10, Seattle, WA 98103, Phone: 206-634-1903, Fax: 206-634-0115, E-mail: cpsdv@cpsdv.org.

Rape Abuse and Incest National Network (RAINN) (see "Hotlines" for further information). Address: 635-B Pennsylvania Avenue SE, Washington, DC 20003, Phone: 1-800-656-HOPE (4673) ext. 3, Fax: 202-544-3556, E-mail: rainnmail@aol.com, Website: www.rainn.org.

Sexual Assault Resource Service (SARS) is designed for nursing professionals involved in providing evaluations of sexually abused victims. SARS' website provides information and technical assistance to individuals and institutions interested in developing new SANE-SART programs or improving existing ones. Website: www.sane-sart.com.

Sexual Assault Information Page (SAIP) is a nonprofit information and referral service. SAIP provides information concerning acquaintance rape, child sexual abuse/assault, incest, rape, ritual abuse, sexual assault, and sexual harassment. Website: http://www.lawguru.com/search/sexassault.html

Additional Abuse And Violence Resources

American Bar Association
740 15th Street, NW
Washington, DC 20005
Phone: 202-662-1000
Website: http://www.abanet.org

American Humane
2007 15th Street N, Suite 201
Arlington, VA 22201
Phone: 303-792-9900
Fax: 703-294-4853
Website: http://
www.americanhumane.org

Child Welfare Information Gateway
Children's Bureau/ACYF
1250 Maryland Avenue, SW
Eighth Floor
Washington, DC 20024
Toll Free: 800-394-3366
Phone: 703-385-7565
Fax: 703-385-3206
Website: http://
www.childwelfare.gov
E-mail: info@childwelfare.gov

Internet Crimes Against Children (ICAC) Task Force Program

Office of Juvenile Justice and
Delinquency Prevention
Office of Justice Programs
U.S. Department of Justice
810 Seventh Street NW
Washington, DC 20531
Phone: 202-307-5911
Website: http://
www.ojjdp.ncjrs.gov/programs/
ProgSummary.asp?pi=3#Resources

Kempe

1825 Marion Street
Denver, CO 80218
Phone: 303-864-5300
Website: http://www.kempe.org

National Center for Missing and Exploited Children

Charles B. Wang International
Children's Building
699 Prince Street
Alexandria, VA 22314
Toll Free: 800-THE-LOST
(800-843-5678)
Phone: 703-274-3900
Fax: 703-274-2200
Website: http://www.ncmec.org
Website: http://www.cybertipline.com

Prevent Child Abuse America

500 N. Michigan Ave., Suite 200
Chicago, IL 60611
Phone: 312-663-3520
Fax: 312-939-8962
Website: http://
www.preventchildabuse.org
E-mail:
mailbox@preventchildabuse.org

Chapter 53

Victims Of Abuse And Violence: Where To Go For Help

The following organizations are among many that have information on child abuse and neglect. Inclusion on this list is for information purposes and does not constitute an endorsement by the Child Welfare Information Gateway or Children's Bureau. For the most current information, please refer to the National Organizations section of the Child Welfare Information Gateway at http://www.childwelfare.gov/organizations/index.cfm.

Recommended updates and additions to the Information Gateway Organization database can be e-mailed to: OrganizationUpdates@childwelfare.gov.

Child Abuse

Childhelp
Phone: 800-4-A-CHILD (800-422-4453)
Who They Help: Child abuse victims, parents, concerned individuals

About This Chapter: Information in this chapter is from "Toll-Free Crisis Hotline Numbers," Child Welfare Information Gateway (www.childwelfare.gov), Children's Bureau, Administration for Children, Youth and Families, U.S. Department of Health and Human Services, January 2007. All contact information was verified in May 2007.

Child Sexual Abuse

Stop It Now!
Phone: 888-PREVENT (888-773-8368)
Who They Help: Child sexual abuse victims, parents, offenders, and concerned individuals

Family Violence

National Domestic Violence Hotline
Phone: 800-799-SAFE (800-799-7233)
Who They Help: Children, parents, friends, and offenders

Missing/Abducted Children

Child Find Of America
Phone: 800-I-AM-LOST (800-426-5678)
Who They Help: Parents reporting lost or abducted children

Child Find Of America: Mediation
Phone: 800-A-WAY-OUT (800-292-9688)
Who They Help: Parents (abduction, prevention, child custody issues)

Child Quest International Sighting Line
Phone: 888-818-HOPE (888-818-4673)
Who They Help: Individuals with missing child emergencies and/or sighting information; victims of abduction

National Center For Missing And Exploited Children
Phone: 800-THE-LOST (800-843-5678)
Who They Help: Families and professionals (social services, law enforcement)

Operation Lookout National Center For Missing Youth
Phone: 800-LOOKOUT (800-566-5688)
Who They Help: Individuals with missing child emergencies and/or sighting information (for children ages 18 and under)

Rape/Incest

Rape And Incest National Network
Phone: 800-656-HOPE; Ext. 1 (800-656-4673; Ext. 1)
Who They Help: Rape and incest victims, media, policy makers, and concerned individuals

Relief For Caregivers

National Respite Locator Service
Phone: 800-677-1116
Who They Help: Parents, caregivers, and professionals caring for children and adults with disabilities, terminal illnesses, or those at risk of abuse or neglect

Youth In Trouble/Runaways

Girls And Boys Town
Phone: 800-448-3000
Who They Help: Abused, abandoned, and neglected girls and boys; parents; family members

Covenant House Hotline
Phone: 800-999-9999
Who They Help: Problem teens and homeless runaways (ages 21 and under), family members, youth substance abusers

National Runaway Switchboard
Phone: 800-RUNAWAY
Who They Help: Runaway and homeless youth, families

National Youth Crisis Hotline
(Youth Development International)
Phone: 800-HIT-HOME (800-448-4663)
Who They Help: Individuals wishing to obtain help for runaways; youth (ages 12 to 18) experiencing drug abuse, teen pregnancy, homelessness, prostitution, or physical, emotional, or sexual abuse

Crime Victims

National Center For Victims Of Crime
Phone: 800-FYI-CALL (800-394-2255)
Who They Help: Families, communities, and individuals harmed by crime

Chapter 54

How And Where To Report Child Abuse

Get Help Now

Call the Childhelp National Child Abuse Hotline at 1-800-4-A-CHILD.

The Childhelp National Child Abuse Hotline is available 24 hours a day, 7 days a week.

A lot of people don't realize it, but every day in the United States thousands of kids are abused and neglected. That adds up to millions of kids each year.

Often children and teens are abused or neglected by the people who are closest to them like family, friends, sitters, neighbors, and sometimes even teachers and coaches. These are the very people that children should feel the safest with.

If you need help or have questions about child abuse or child neglect, call the Childhelp National Child Abuse Hotline at 1-800-4-A-CHILD (1-800-422-4453) then push "1" to talk to a counselor.

About This Chapter: Information in this chapter, "Get Help Now" and "What to Expect when Calling," is reprinted with permission from Childhelp®. © 2006 Childhelp. All rights reserved. To Get Help, call the Childhelp National Child Abuse Hotline at 1-800-4-A-CHILD. To Give Help, visit www.childhelp.org. Additional information under the heading "Other Child Abuse Reporting Numbers" is from the Child Welfare Information Gateway (www.childwelfare.gov). All contact information was verified in May 2007.

The Hotline counselors are there 365 days a year to help kids and adults who are worried about kids they suspect are being abused or neglected. You can call this number if you live in the United States, Canada, Puerto Rico, Guam, or the U.S. Virgin Islands.

The call is free and anonymous. (The Hotline counselors don't know who you are, and you don't have to tell them.) There won't be a charge for the call on your telephone bill if you use a regular phone or a pay phone. If you use a mobile phone or cell phone, there may be a charge, and it may show up on the telephone bill. Don't use a mobile or cell phone if you want to be sure your call is a secret, but please do not make prank calls to the Hotline. This will tie up the phones and keep us from talking to someone who really needs help right away.

What To Expect When Calling

When calling for information on reporting child abuse, a recorded message will tell you to press or say "1" to talk to a Hotline crisis counselor. This is the option to choose if you have one of the following situations:

- need help and want to talk to a counselor

- have questions about child abuse or want to know where to go for information on reporting child abuse, to report suspected or known abuse in your community, or want a referral to an agency near you

The recording will give you these two other options:

- **Press 3** if you want literature mailed to you. (Allow two weeks for delivery via the U.S. Postal Service.)

- **Press 2** if you want to make a donation to Childhelp.

When you select option "1", a counselor will answer and say "Childhelp crisis counselor. How may I help you?" If the person calling speaks a language other than English, the Hotline counselor will set up a three-way call with a translator.

The counselor will do the following:

- listen to your concerns and needs

- answer your questions

- ask you questions to be sure he or she understands what you are saying

- suggest things you can do to get help

- provide referrals utilizing a database of thousands of emergency, social service, and support resources located in the United States and Canada

If you are a child or teen who is in danger, the Hotline counselor will help you contact someone such as Child Protective Services or the police. If needed, the Hotline counselor will stay on the phone as part of a three-way call.

The Hotline counselor will not tape the telephone conversation or ask for your name (unless you ask to have literature mailed to you).

Other Child Abuse Reporting Numbers

The following organizations are among many that have information on child abuse reporting numbers. Inclusion on this list is for information purposes and does not constitute an endorsement by Child Welfare Information Gateway or the Children's Bureau. For the most current information, please refer to the National Organizations section of Child Welfare Information Gateway at http://www.childwelfare.gov/organizations/index.cfm.

Alabama
Local (toll): 334-242-9500
Website: http://www.dhr.state.al.us
Click on "Services," then click on "Child Protective Services."

Alaska
Toll Free: 800-478-4444 (AK calls only)
Website: http://www.hss.state.ak.us/ocs/default.htm

Arizona
Toll Free: 888-SOS-CHILD (888-767-2445)
Website: http://www.de.state.az.us/dcyf/cmdps/cps/default.asp

Arkansas
Toll Free: 800-482-5964
http://www.state.ar.us/dhs/chilnfam/child_protective_services.htm

California
Website: http://www.dss.cahwnet.gov
Use the site's search feature to search for "Child Protective Services," then click on the link identified as "Social Services-Main Web-Child Protective Services." Use the website above for information on reporting or call Childhelp® (800-422-4453) for assistance.

Colorado
Local (toll): 303-866-5932
Website: http://www.cdhs.state.co.us/childwelfare/FAQ.htm

Connecticut
Toll Free: 800-842-2288
TDD: 800-624-5518
Website: http://www.state.ct.us/dcf/HOTLINE.htm

Delaware
Toll Free: 800-292-9582
Website: http://www.state.de.us/kids

District Of Columbia
Local (toll): 202-671-SAFE (202-671-7233)
Website: http://cfsa.dc.gov
Click on "Child Protective Services," then "How to Report Child Abuse."

Florida
Toll Free: 800-96-ABUSE (800-962-2873)
Website: http://www.dcf.state.fl.us/abuse

Georgia
Website: http://dfcs.dhr.georgia.gov/portal/site
Click on the website above for information on reporting or call Childhelp® (800-422-4453) for assistance.

Hawaii
Local (toll): 808-832-5300
Website: http://www.hawaii.gov/dhs/protection/social_services/child_welfare

Idaho

Toll Free: 800-926-2588

Website: http://www.healthandwelfare.idaho.gov

Click on "Site Map," then "Children," then "Child Protection."

Illinois

Toll Free: 800-252-2873 (IL calls only)

Local (toll): 217-524-2606

Website: http://www.state.il.us/dcfs/child/index.shtml

Indiana

Toll Free: 800-800-5556

Website: http://www.in.gov/dcs/protection/dfcchi.html

Iowa

Toll Free: 800-362-2178

Website: http://www.dhs.state.ia.us

Click on "Report Child Abuse."

Kansas

Toll Free: 800-922-5330 (KS calls only)

Website: http://www.srskansas.org/services/child_protective_services.htm

Kentucky

Toll Free: 800-752-6200

Website: http://www.pcaky.org

Louisiana

Website: http://www.dss.state.la.us

Click on "Report Child Abuse/Neglect."

Use the website above for information on reporting or call Childhelp®
(800-422-4453) for assistance.

Maine

Toll Free: 800-452-1999

TTY: 800-963-9490

Website: http://www.maine.gov/dhhs/bcfs/abusereporting.htm

Maryland
Website: http://www.dhr.state.md.us/cps/report.htm
Use the website above for information on reporting or call Childhelp®
(800-422-4453) for assistance.

Massachusetts
Toll Free: 800-792-5200
Website: http://www.mass.gov
Click on "Site Map." Under "Family," click on "Domestic Violence &
Abuse," then "Child Abuse and Domestic Violence." Next, click on "Child
Abuse and Neglect," then "Reporting Child Abuse and Neglect."

Michigan
Website: http://www.michigan.gov
Click on "Education & Children's Services," then "Children's Services."
Next, click on "Child Care & Safety," then "Report Suspected Child
Neglect/Abuse." Then click on "Complaint Process."
Use the website above for information on reporting or call Childhelp®
(800-422-4453) for assistance.

Minnesota
Website: http://www.dhs.state.mn.us
Click on "Children," then "Child protection."
Use the website above for information on reporting or call Childhelp®
(800-422-4453) for assistance.

Mississippi
Toll Free: 800-222-8000 (MS calls only)
Local (toll): 601-359-4991
Website: http://www.mdhs.state.ms.us/fcs_prot.html

Missouri
Toll Free: 800-392-3738
Local (toll): 573-751-3448
Website: http://www.dss.mo.gov/cd/rptcan.htm

Montana
Toll Free: 866-820-5437
Website: http://www.dphhs.mt.gov/aboutus/divisions/childfamilyservices/index.shtml

Nebraska
Toll Free: 800-652-1999
Website: http://www.hhs.state.ne.us/cha/chaindex.htm

Nevada
Toll Free: 800-992-5757
Local (toll): 775-684-4400
Website: http://dcfs.state.nv.us/DCFS_PhDirectory.htm

New Hampshire
Toll Free: 800-894-5533
Local (toll): 603-271-6556
Website: http://www.dhhs.state.nh.us/DHHS/BCP/default.htm

New Jersey
Toll Free: 877-652-2873
TDD: 800-835-5510
TTY: 800-835-5510
Website: http://www.state.nj.us/humanservices/dyfs/hotlines.html

New Mexico
Toll Free: 800-797-3260
Local (toll): 505-841-6100
Website: http://www.cyfd.org/index.htm

New York
Toll Free: 800-342-3720
Local (toll): 518-474-8740
TDD: 800-369-2437
Website: http://www.ocfs.state.ny.us/main/cps

North Carolina

Website: http://www.dhhs.state.nc.us/dss/cps/index.htm
Use the website above for information on reporting or call Childhelp®
(800-422-4453) for assistance.

North Dakota

Website: http://www.nd.gov/dhs/services/childfamily/cps/#reporting
Use the website above for information on reporting or call Childhelp®
(800-422-4453) for assistance.

Ohio

Website: http://jfs.ohio.gov/county/cntydir.stm
Contact the county Public Children Services Agency using the list on the
above website or call Childhelp USA® (800-422-4453) for assistance.

Oklahoma

Toll Free: 800-522-3511
Website: http://www.okdhs.org/programsandservices/cps

Oregon

Website: http://www.oregon.gov/DHS/children/abuse/cps/report.shtml
Use the website above for information on reporting or call Childhelp®
(800-422-4453) for assistance.

Pennsylvania

Toll Free: 800-932-0313
Website: http://www.dpw.state.pa.us/Child/ChildAbuseNeglect

Puerto Rico

Toll Free: 800-981-8333
Local (toll): 787-749-1333
Spanish Information Website: http://www.gobierno.pr/GPRPortal/
StandAlone/AgencyInformation.aspx?Filter=177

Rhode Island

Toll Free: 800-RI-CHILD (800-742-4453)
Website: http://www.dcyf.ri.gov
Click on "Child Welfare."

South Carolina
Local (toll): 803-898-7318
Website: http://www.state.sc.us/dss/cps/index.html

South Dakota
Local (toll): 605-773-3227
Website: http://www.state.sd.us/social/CPS/Services/offices.htm

Tennessee
Toll Free: 877-237-0004
Website: http://www.tennessee.gov/youth/childsafety.htm

Texas
Toll Free: 800-252-5400
Website: https://www.dfps.state.tx.us
Click on "Child Protective Services," then "How to Report Abuse."

Utah
Toll Free: 800-678-9399
Website: http://www.hsdcfs.utah.gov

Vermont
After hours: 800-649-5285 (VT calls only)
Website: http://www.dcf.state.vt.us/fsd/reporting/index.html

Virginia
Toll Free: 800-552-7096
Local (toll): 804-786-8536
Website: http://www.dss.virginia.gov/family/cps/index.html

Washington
Toll Free: 866-END-HARM (866-363-4276)
After hours: 800-562-5624
TTY: 800-624-6186
Website: http://www.dshs.wa.gov
Click on "DSHS services." Under "Abuse & Neglect," then under "Child, Reporting," click on "Child Abuse and Neglect Reporting (CA)."

West Virginia
Toll Free: 800-352-6513
Website: http://www.wvdhhr.org/bcf/children_adult/cps/report.asp

Wisconsin
Website: http://www.dhfs.state.wi.us/Children/CPS/cpswimap.HTM
Use the website above for information on reporting or call Childhelp®
(800-422-4453) for assistance.

Wyoming
Website: http://dfsweb.state.wy.us/menu.htm
Use the website above for information on reporting or call Childhelp®
(800-422-4453) for assistance.

Chapter 55

Additional Reading About Abuse And Violence

Books

Bullying: How to Deal with Taunting, Teasing, and Tormenting

Kathleen Winkler; Enslow Publishers, Berkeley Heights, NJ
August 2005. ISBN: 978-0766023550

Date Violence

Elaine Landau; Franklin Watts, London, England
March 2005. ISBN: 978-0531166130

Family and Friends' Guide to Domestic Violence: How to Listen, Talk and Take Action When Someone You Care About is Being Abused

Elaine Weiss, Ed. D; Volcano Press, Volcano, CA
October 2003. ISBN: 978-1884244223

About This Chapter: This chapter includes a compilation of various resources from many sources deemed reliable. It serves as a starting point for further research and is not intended to be comprehensive. Inclusion does not constitute endorsement. Resources in this chapter are categorized by type and, under each type, they are listed alphabetically by title to make topics easier to identify.

Fear Less: Real Truth about Risk, Safety, and Security in a Time of Terrorism
Gavin de Becker; Little, Brown and Company, New York, NY
January 2002. ISBN: 978-0316085960

High School Hazing: When Rites Become Wrongs
Hank Nuwer; Franklin Watts, London, England
September 2000. ISBN: 978-0531164655

How Long Does It Hurt: A Guide to Recovering from Incest and Sexual Abuse for Teenagers, Their Friends, and Their Families
Cynthia L. Mather and Kristina E. Debye; Jossey-Bass, San Francisco, CA
November 2004. ISBN: 978-0787975692

How to Stop a Stalker
Mike Proctor; Prometheus Books, Amherst, NY
August 2003. ISBN: 978-1591020912

In Love and In Danger: A Teen's Guide to Breaking Free of Abusive Relationships
Barrie Levy; Seal Press, Emeryville, CA
September 2006. ISBN: 978-1580051873

Internet Safety
Josepha Sherman; Franklin Watts, London, England
September 2003. ISBN: 978-0531162125

Invisible Girls: The Truth about Sexual Abuse
Patti Feuereisen; Seal Press, Emeryville, CA
March 2005. ISBN: 978-1580051354

Kids Helping Kids Break the Silence of Sexual Abuse
Linda Lee Foltz; Lighthouse Point Press, Pittsburgh, PA
March 2003. ISBN: 978-0963796684

Live Aware, Not in Fear: The 411 After 9-11
Donna K. Wells and Bruce C. Morris; Health Communications, Inc.,
Deerfield Beach, FL
February 2002. ISBN: 978-0757300134

Respect: A Girl's Guide to Getting Respect & Dealing When Your Line Is Crossed
Courtney Macavinta and Andrea Vander Pluym; Free Spirit Publishing,
Minneapolis, MN
September 2005. ISBN: 978-1575421773

A Safe Place: Beyond Sexual Abuse
Jan Morrison; Waterbrook Press, Colorado Springs, CO
May 2002. ISBN: 978-0877887478

Safe Teen: Powerful Alternatives to Violence
Anita Roberts; Raincoast Books, Vancouver, British Columbia
February 2001. ISBN: 978-1896095998

School Violence: Deadly Lessons
Francha Roffe Menhard; Enslow Publishers, Berkeley Heights, NJ
July 2000. ISBN: 978-0766013582

Self-Injury: When Pain Feels Good
Edward T. Welch; P & R Publishing Company, Phillipsburg, NJ
March 2004. ISBN: 978-0875526973

Unmasking Sexual Con Games: A Teen's Guide to Avoiding Emotional Grooming and Dating Violence
Kathleen M. McGee and Laura J. Buddenberg; Boys Town Press, Boys Town, NE
February 2003. ISBN: 978-1889322551

When Nothing Matters Anymore: A Survival Guide for Depressed Teens
Bev Cobain; Free Spirit Publishing, Minneapolis, MN
April 2007. ISBN: 978-1575422350

Youth Gangs: Terror in Our Streets

Janet Butler with B. J. Mayeur; Infinity Publishing, West Conshohocken, PA
April 2003. ISBN: 978-0741413468

Articles

"Adolescent Self-Injury Can Be Cured," *United Press International*, September 2, 2003, p1008245w2003.

"Breaking Free: After Overcoming Her Boyfriend's Abuse, Shaina Weisbrot Has Made It Her Mission to Stop Relationship Violence Among Teens," by Leah Paulos, *Scholastic Choices*, February-March 2007 v22 i5, p. 10(6).

"Bullying Puts Students in a Dangerous, Catch-22 Position," by Melissa Vargas, *Fort Worth Star-Telegram*, November 21, 2006, p. NA.

"Dangerous Liaisons: Dating Is Supposed to Be Fun, Right? Not If Your Crush Is a Control Freak. Or Worse," by Christina Alex, *Girls' Life*, April-May 2007 v13 i5, p. 64(3).

"Domestic Violence: Women at Increasing Risk from Batterers with Firearms; Firearms 'Triple Threat' to Women Says Former Prosecutor," *US Newswire*, May 25, 2006, p. NA.

"50,000 Americans Touched by Domestic Violence Programs in a Single Day," *US Newswire*, March 13, 2007, p. NA.

"For Your Protection," *Current Health 2*, a *Weekly Reader* publication, March 2007 v33 i7, p. 6(2).

"The Games Kids Play: Are Mature Video Games Too Violent for Teens," *Current Events*, a *Weekly Reader* publication, February 7, 2003 v102 i18, p. 3(1).

"Is There a Relationship Between Victim and Partner Alcohol Use During an Intimate Partner Violence Event? Findings from an Urban Emergency Department Study of Abused Women," by Sherry Lipsky, Raul Caetano, Craig A. Field, and Gregory L. Larkin, *Journal of Studies on Alcohol*, May 2005 v66 i3, p. 407(6).

"Laws Shield Pets from Domestic Violence," by Emily Bazar, *USA Today*, August 24, 2006, p. 03A.

"Psychopathologic Behavior: A Consequence of Bullying," by Karl E. Miller, *American Family Physician*, January 15, 2007 v75 i2, p. 252.

"Recognizing Domestic Partner Abuse," *Harvard Women's Health Watch*, September 2006, p. NA.

"Safe Surfing: Millions of Teens Spend Hours on the Internet. If You're One of Them, Here's How to Protect Yourself from Online Predators," by Libby Tucker, *Scholastic Choices*, September 2006 v22 i1, p. 6(6).

"Self-Injury: The Secret Language of Pain for Teenagers," by Len Austin and Julie Kortum, *Education*, Spring 2004 v124 i3, p. 517(11).

"Sex and Drug Use Increase Teen Suicide Risk," *Obesity, Fitness & Wellness Week*, October 2, 2004, p. 345.

"Sibling Maltreatment: The Forgotten Abuse," by Mark S. Kiselica and Mandy Morrill-Richards, *Journal of Counseling and Development*, Spring 2007 v85 i2, p. 148(14).

"Stalker Usually Not a Stranger; Trigger Is Often Jealousy," by Wendy Koch, *USA Today*, February 9, 2007, p. 04A.

"Working Teens Increasingly Victims of Sexual Harassment," *Obesity, Fitness & Wellness Week*, June 12, 2004, p. 28.

Index

Index

Page numbers that appear in *Italics* refer to illustrations. Page numbers that have a small 'n' after the page number refer to information shown as Notes at the beginning of each chapter. Page numbers that appear in **Bold** refer to information contained in boxes on that page (except Notes information at the beginning of each chapter).